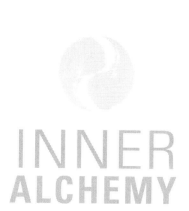

INNER
ALCHEMY

ALSO BY PEDRAM SHOJAI

The Urban Monk: Eastern Wisdom and Modern Hacks to Stop Time and Find Success, Happiness, and Peace

The Art of Stopping Time: Practical Mindfulness for Busy People

THE **URBAN MONK'S GUIDE** TO
HAPPINESS, HEALTH & VITALITY

INNER
ALCHEMY

PEDRAM SHOJAI, OMD

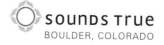

SOUNDS TRUE
BOULDER, COLORADO

Sounds True
Boulder, CO 80306

Published 2019

Previously published as *Rise and Shine: Awaken Your Energy Body with Taoist Alchemy and Qi Gong*, 2011.

This book is not intended as a substitute for the medical recommendations of physicians or other health-care providers. Rather, it is intended to offer information to help the reader cooperate with physicians and health-care providers in a mutual quest for optimal well-being. We advise readers to carefully review and understand the ideas presented and to seek the advice of a qualified professional before attempting to use them.

Cover design by Lisa Kerans
Book design by Beth Skelley

Printed in Canada

Library of Congress Cataloging-in-Publication Data

Names: Shojai, Pedram, author.
Title: Inner alchemy : the urban monk's guide to happiness, health, and
    vitality / Pedram Shojai.
Description: Boulder, CO : Sounds True, Inc., 2019. | Includes
    bibliographical references.
Identifiers: LCCN 2018006716 (print) | LCCN 2018040627 (ebook) |
    ISBN 9781683642046 (ebook) | ISBN 9781683641674 (pbk.)
Subjects: LCSH: Alchemy–Religious aspects–Taoism. | Qi gong.
Classification: LCC BL1923 (ebook) | LCC BL1923 .S575 2019 (print) |
    DDC 299.5/1444–dc23
LC record available at https://lccn.loc.gov/2018006716

10 9 8 7 6 5 4 3 2 1

CONTENTS

LIST OF FIGURES

LIST OF TABLES

INTRODUCTION

I have learned that there is no spirituality higher than our own enlightened humanity. The joys of the human experience, once we are awake, are the most incredible gifts we have been given, and this is what I am here to impart. *Inner Alchemy* tells the story of the incredible teachings of Taoist alchemy and the practice of energy work called qi gong—and it does it in plain English.

In this book, you will learn how to read and clear your energy field, to open to the inner language of your body, and to access your subconscious mind. All of this will allow you to connect to and communicate with Source energy, which is already always flowing through you. This is how you turn the "lead" of your day-to-day life into "gold" so you can be healthier, happier, and, ultimately, of service to others and the planet.

I am the juxtaposition of many traditions and cultures, and I am here to hold the center. I found tai chi when I was in the pre-med program at the University of California, Los Angeles. From there, I learned kung fu and qi gong and eventually became a Taoist monk and a doctor of oriental medicine. While I was in the high Himalayas, I realized I needed to be back in the world. Now I'm a householder with a wife and kids. I'm the founder of well.org, I make movies, and I have a large business, The Urban Monk, which was born out of my folly—trying to get busy, urban, working people to try the powerful alchemical stuff that has helped me. Unless you are living in a monastery, you don't have an hour and a half for yoga and then two hours to meditate, plus time for a salt bath soak; living as a traditional monk is a difficult yet privileged lifestyle that renounces the world. My focus for the past twenty years has been to bring what I learned on the mountain down to the city.

Although originally written prior to my book *The Urban Monk*, the content here complements and builds upon the concepts and practices there. This book was written when I was more "monk" and less "urban." It covers the heavy stuff that is the basis of all the spiritual talk out there. My goal is to have this book serve as a gateway text that introduces alchemical principles and inspires you to develop a steadfast personal practice. In this book, I give you all the necessary tools you need in order to start. I've taken out the fluff to offer a "deep dive" into the core teachings that have been lost by the mainstream. We can't throw the baby out with the bathwater, and this book is "the baby."

My task at hand here is to demystify much of this information and bring it down to earth. I chose to study Taoism because it stands for balance. It teaches us to balance all aspects of our lives and to bring harmony to the material and the spiritual. It breaks up the division in our way of thinking, allowing us to become whole again.

My promise to you is that if you practice what you learn in this book, your life will change in ways you have never imagined. Let me be very clear about something, though: I am not the one doing this for you. I am not interested in being a guru or getting nailed to a cross. *You* are the only one who can wake yourself up. I am providing you with the tools and support. My interest is in your growth and your personal development. I know these techniques work because they have worked for me and for many thousands before me. They have helped me wake up, and they will do the same for you if you practice them.

In part I of this book, I lay out the philosophy and background needed to gain a basic understanding of the body's energy matrix and the nature of the challenges you currently face. In part II, I provide specific exercises and techniques that are designed to clean your energy field and wake you up. This includes instruction in diet, exercise, sleep, and basic lifestyle modifications. In part III, I offer more advanced techniques and lay out a formula for you to practice so you can literally change your life within a hundred days. You can find free videos for two of the exercises at SoundsTrue.com/inner-alchemy/bonus, and there are many more resources on my websites, well.org and theurbanmonk.com. In this part of the book, I have also laid out the baseline knowledge and tools you need in order to clean up and refine your energy. I get into the most profound work I have ever experienced in my years of training. This information is your birthright; deep down, you already know most of it. I am just here to remind you and to hold your hand until you are ready to shine like a star.

I constantly strive for balance in my life, and I have a pretty broad range; this is also true for my writing style. Sometimes you will get the monk; at other times, you will get the monkey. Both are me, and both are important. I am here to humanize this process and make it joyful. I will, at times, speak of things that seem very far out there and very strange, but I'm not asking you to believe everything I have to say—yet. Actually, go ahead and read this book as fiction if you'd like and just see where your mind takes you later. In fact, I don't expect anyone to believe *anything*. Put the principles you learn in this book into practice, try the exercises, and see for yourself. Only you can awaken you, and the *experience* of the Divine supersedes any belief in abstract concepts taught through ancient books.

Additionally, I find it important to note that you will be introduced to a variety of subjects in this book that draw from various traditions. Although I am a Taoist teacher primarily, I also have training in Western esotericism, Buddhism, Kabala, medicine, herbalism, and a whole host of self-help techniques from various schools. I regularly draw from what I find useful in order to make the content more accessible. If you are looking for the work of a Taoist purist, then this book may not be for you. I believe that we are living in a time of experimentalism and that the postmodern era has led us into the deconstruction of the cultural barriers of the past. You don't have to be Chinese to study kung fu and be good at it. Likewise, you don't need to wear a turban to practice yoga. As a matter of fact, please just be yourself and wake up. You are perfect just as you are!

You are about to embark on a journey. Along the way, you will learn a great many things and discover facets of yourself that have been hiding right under your nose. There's a lot of heavy stuff here, but nothing is heavier than your own shadow. The hardest challenge you'll face in this process is being honest with yourself and opening to the reality of your situation. This is the real spiritual work. You cannot refine lead until you pick it up and weigh it. You cannot talk about some far-off concept unless you have experienced it within your own flesh. In the course of this book, you are going to walk through a variety of topics and learn a great deal about yourself. Why should you do this? What's in it for you? Everything! You are the only one who can liberate yourself from the prison of your perceived limitations. There is unlimited peace, power, freedom, money, love, and joy right on the other side of letting go of your stories and waking up to your true potential. There is no real darkness once you come home to yourself; there is no darkness to fear, and your higher self knows this. Tap into your Source energy and wake up to the adventure life has in store for you.

Enjoy the book and do the work—you'll be happy you did!

In loving light,
Pedram Shojai

PART I

TAOIST ALCHEMICAL SCIENCE

1

THE FREE FLOW OF ENERGY

All the power that ever was or will be is here now.

HERMES TRISMEGISTUS, The Pattern on the Trestleboard

The human mind is infinite. And because of the vastness of our comprehension, we all have certain blind spots in our awareness. They
may manifest in the unconscious tone we take when our father
rings on the phone or maybe in the rush to smoke a cigarette when we
feel overwhelmed. Maybe they appear as the nervous things we say when
put into a challenging situation, or perhaps they are what allow us to
go through an entire workday and not know what happened, simply
moving through the motions all day long. Most of us can also relate to
getting lost in social media, not realizing what time it is and being late
for something important. Regardless of the item, we have all faced things
that rear their ugly heads out of our subconscious mind. We don't feel
fully in control and can sense a powerful battery of stored-up emotions
and grievances haunting us from our past. This has become the condition of most of us human beings every day of our lives. We struggle with
our internal dialogue and push as best we can to get through our days
and make our lives go around. *It doesn't have to be this way.*

There is a way to escape this vicious cycle and break free of our
mental and spiritual bondage. It is based in an ancient system of Taoist
alchemy that is designed to clear the energy fields around us and bring
balance back to our lives.

This alchemy is the practice of turning our "lead" into "gold." The process of turning the material "lead" of our human experience into the "gold" of spiritual awakening is the essence of this ancient science of spirituality. This sounds interesting in theory; however, to make it a reality requires a deep understanding of energy flow and the internal landscape of the human energy field. This knowledge used to be widely understood on this planet but has slowly contracted into obscure circles in tucked-away monasteries worldwide. We fell asleep to the knowledge of our true nature, but now it is time to wake up. The great secret of alchemy has been preserved for thousands of years, and we are quite fortunate to be living in a time when we can be a part of the great re-dissemination of this ancient information.

To begin the process of awakening, we need a frame of reference—a starting point from which to launch. It is this: our bodies *are* the alchemical vehicles, and our experiences in this world are the proverbial "lead" that will be turned into "gold." Listen to your body. Don't ignore it because you're focusing on some higher spiritual goal; instead, learn to balance your internal energies and harmonize your emotions. This is a very important step in practical spirituality and in living life. A famous alchemical axiom states that heaven is *within* us and not *above* us, as many have mistaken it to be. The exploration of our own consciousness gives us a glimpse at the mind of God. The more we come to understand our true nature, the more we will be able to understand reality. It starts with each of us developing a *personal* understanding of how reality works and how we fit into the picture. To do this, we first need to examine some basic principles in greater depth.

Earth's Energy Fields

According to modern physicists, chaos is the dominant ruling principle of the universe. All things move toward chaos as it governs and tears apart all things that are manifest. Life, in contrast, is an ordered system. In fact, when organic systems start to fall out of order, they begin to experience deterioration, decomposition, mutation (which leads to cancer), and the eventual breakdown of living systems (aging). Our goal as living beings, therefore, is to support, enhance, and harness the power of life and guard it against the annihilation coming from outside. To better understand this, let's look at some basic concepts in biomagnetics. Look at the image of planet Earth in figure 1.1.

The lines coming into each pole represent the edges of the magnetic field generated by the polarity of the planet. This dynamic tension is an important interface between the positive (yang, or south) and negative (yin, or north) poles on the planet, which create an energy field wherein all life can be supported. In fact, fluctuations in this field can be very harmful to all life-forms on Earth. The three-dimensional manifestation, called a *toroidal* field, is the basis of all hyperdimensional physics and energy work.

The distinction between the electric field and the magnetic field is an important one. The magnetic field can be measured by forces acting on certain kinds of materials, such as the element iron. (It is interesting to note that the hemoglobin molecule of our red blood

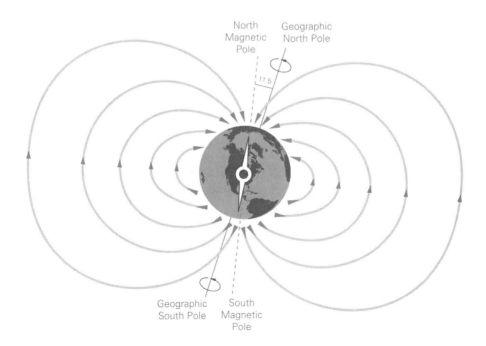

FIGURE 1.1   Earth's Magnetic Field

cells is primarily centered around an iron ion to which the oxygen binds.) The electric field can be measured by forces acting on electrically charged particles, such as sodium and chloride. The electric charge of an object is the sum of the charges of its particles. All nerve and muscle functions in our bodies rely on electrical charge gradients that are constantly shifting. Electrical signaling is therefore the body's internal language of operation. These two fields—electrical and magnetic—always coexist with the same intensity at a given location and instant in time. They are really parts of the same field, which is thus called the *electromagnetic* field.[1]

The importance of the electromagnetic field to our bodies can be illustrated by what happens to us in its absence. One of the problems for early orbiting astronauts was that their biological systems were beginning to break down while *outside* of the Earth's magnetic field; they were feeling sick and weak for no apparent reason—at least, no reason apparent to us. The scientists working on the Soviet space program figured out why this was happening and then shared their findings with NASA scientists, who eventually found a way to mimic the earth's magnetic field using a frequency called the Schumann resonance. They can now create energy field bubbles for astronauts who are performing outer-space missions.

The lowest frequency (and highest intensity) mode of the Schumann resonance occurs at a frequency of approximately 7.83 Hz, which is just under eight cycles per second. This frequency happens to coincide with the alpha rhythm of our brain waves, which is the frequency closest to the state of meditation and deep connection with our surroundings. Everything tunes to vibrations. In physics, there are particles and waves, both of which seem to have an underlying system of communication we are just starting to understand. The frequency-based phenomena all revolve around waveform. Our bodies can detect and respond to waves of energy just as our ears can distinguish different sounds from waves in the auditory spectrum. There is a resonant vibration with all light, sound, and movement, and these are some of the energies we can sense with our hands and within people's fields. These particles, or photons, seem to travel through our bodies and trigger a light-based system of interaction between the DNA molecules in our cells. These light particles apparently have something to do with how the DNA zips and unzips in its transcoding of information.[2] This knowledge may give us some hints at how the ancients were able to decipher the language of the "coiled serpents" and hear the song of Creation when looking inward (refer to further discussion on this in part III). The flow of energy becomes the fundamental currency for the field of life, which lives in a perpetual array of fields within fields—all the way up to the scale of the entire universe and down to the smallest subatomic particles we can find.

Dynamo theory explains that Earth's magnetic field is caused not by magnetized iron deposits but mostly by electric currents in the planet's liquid outer core. The convection of molten iron within this outer core, along with a Coriolis effect caused by the overall planetary rotation, tends to organize these electric currents in rolls aligned along the north-south polar axis. When conducting fluid flows across an existing magnetic field, electric currents are induced, which in turn create another magnetic field. When this magnetic field reinforces the original magnetic field, it creates a self-sustaining dynamo. The dynamo theory, which explains how the Earth's magnetic field is reinforced,[3] is a very important concept in our internal cultivation, because the dynamic flow of blood and *qi* energy within our bodies forms a microcosm of this same dynamo phenomenon. This theory explains why the smooth flow of energy within the body is vitally important to the integrity of our energy fields. It is almost as if our blood is a microcosm of the molten core flowing inside the planet—both working to generate and reinforce the energy field around the external "body."

These fields are the foundation of all life. They create a dynamic flow and allow for living systems to exist within them. Each living system has its own energy field that supports the living cells within it, all the way down to the subatomic level and all the way up to a universal level. We are fields of life within one great field, all dependent upon each other and all mutually enhancing the ability of others to grow.[4] We affect the Earth's field with our consciousness, just as the Earth's changes in field strength affect us daily. The interconnection of the fields of energy throughout the universe creates an environment where a fluctuation in *any* energy field will resonate and affect all other energy fields in the entire universe. This nonlocal influence seems to cross both space and time and is becoming the subject of much debate in the world of physics.

The ancient sages knew this to be true because they *experienced it* through meditations and their knowledge of how their own energy fields operated. Being able to sense these things became the fundamental mark of a true gnostic, or a person who found the answers within him- or herself and, because of this, was able to unlock the secrets of the universe. The concepts imparted in this book come from a vast body of knowledge that has been confirmed by hundreds of ascended masters over thousands of years. They found these answers internally and were able to agree on the principles they discovered. They were able to feel the energy running through their bodies and to track its flow through the various organs. They represent an age-old living tradition of seekers who have learned to *be* the very knowledge they were seeking. These masters learned about the secrets of our luminous bodies and developed an impressive understanding of energy fields well before we had developed any instruments to measure such phenomena with our modern technology.

The Human Energy Field

As a human being, you have a positive "yang" pole at the top of your head and a negative "yin" pole in your perineum (the base of the spine), as well as smaller yin poles at the bottoms of the feet that dip a couple of feet into the ground. The poles create an energy field around your body, with internal "stars" along the spine contained within. These concentrations of energy cascade down like the descending colors of a prism or a rainbow, beginning with white, moving to violet, and going all the way down to red at the base. These internal "stars," which are called *chakras* in the Indian tradition and *dantiens* in the Chinese tradition, represent the areas where the energy of all Creation is differentiated from the crown, which is the highest vibration, down to the root center, which is the densest or most earthly vibration (see figure 1.2). The goal is not to ignore the base centers and run to the crown; rather, it is to bring peace, understanding, awareness, and, most important, *balance* to each of these centers.

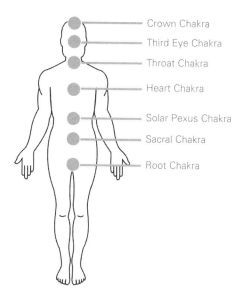

FIGURE 1.2   Human Energy Centers (Chakras)

The harmonious flow of our energy field enhances life and nourishes the brain and internal organs. Any problems with this flow, or *impedance*, cause breakdowns in this network and lead to ailments on the physical, mental, emotional, and spiritual levels, all of which are reflections or octaves of the same energy. Each chakra represents a different archetypal aspect of the human experience, and many of our life lessons are to be learned by harmonizing these centers. We start by forgiving and healing the wounds and perceived assaults that have driven us to create the defense system we refer to as our "ego." In our ignorance, we take this primitive defense mechanism and apply it to various aspects of our lives, effectively cutting off the free flow of energy available to us. This vital energy flows through *nadi* (Indian) or *meridians* (Chinese), which carry it through the entire body and literally bring life to every cell of the body through a comprehensive network of channels. The scope of this network is beyond this book (many great books on this subject already exist), but it is important to know that any energetic blockage will be reflected somewhere in the body, and it will usually hold a mental and emotional charge with it.

The smooth flow of blood and energy in our body helps make our energy fields dynamic, as their intensity varies with time. The human energy field is an accurate reflection of the inner workings of the physical body and mental processes. In fact, all emotional, spiritual, and physical phenomena will be reflected somewhere in this field. We often feel and see lulls and dips in these fields after meals or with the rise of certain emotional content in our lives. In fact, energetic attachments are often trapped in our fields, blocking the smooth flow of energy throughout our body. Herein rests the core issue.

Unexamined emotions and memories that we are not currently willing to deal with are often the cause of these blockages. So how do they do it? These memories and emotions get stored in our bioelectric field (this includes our physical body, which is simply denser energy) and act as a dam, trapping more energy behind. They await a release, which can be very difficult, as it requires us to focus our attention on the dam with forgiveness and love. A whole chapter of this book is devoted to this concept. For now, know that we accumulate these blockages throughout our lives, and these frozen energies are what cause further suffering today. They cut the vital current of our energy and literally make us weak and sick by reducing the free flow of our energy field.

The good news is that you can learn to detect blockages in your field and use certain exercises and techniques to correct the flow of energy. Once you learn to read the signs in your energy field, you can open yourself to a vast inner language of communication within your body; this inner language has always been going on under the radar, but you've likely been mostly blind to it. In fact, once you get an understanding of this system, you will expose yourself to a sub-conscious mind that has been anxious to communicate with you for years! It has always been sending you signals in the form of tingling hands, hunches, sudden headaches, the chills—essentially whatever it can do to get your attention. Once you learn to finally listen to this internal language, you will begin to complete a powerful circuit of personal communication and connection to Source. It is through your subconscious mind that you will begin to interpret the language of your energy field.

PERSONAL JOURNEYS   Night Vision

When I was in the thick of my martial arts training, my teacher would have us go into the mountains at night during a new moon. We would spend a short time meditating and then go for a walk along the trails. The lesson was to soften the eyes and learn to see the energy fields of the plants around us. At first, the whole thing sounded crazy. It was dark, and I was stumbling around, wondering if I'd ever grasp this pseudo-Jedi nonsense. I kept trying to see with my eyes and was frustrated.

The lesson was to *soften* the eyes because seeing with *shen*, or spirit, requires a more passive form of vision. Slowly, I began to relax into it and started to see "fuzzy stuff" on the tops of the plants. Of course, I thought that my eyes were playing tricks on me and I was just seeing the plants themselves or the reflections of city lights. After a while though, I started to see fluctuations in the patterns of this energy. It was almost like the fields shifted as I approached, in an acknowledgment of approaching life-forms.

I conducted this training for many moons until the vision of energy fields of living things became commonplace for me. I could then start to see the energy in the daytime as well. It is incredible to see how powerful an energy field looks in undisturbed nature as opposed to in a city setting. It is as if all the life energy synergistically comes together to compound into a bigger field. I started to see the distinct energy fields of forests and mountainsides, while a particular valley would be alight with its own unique "vibe," and I would watch the energy shift throughout.

I then started seeing the same phenomenon in people—when they would come in contact with certain people or groups of people, their fields would grow and get stronger. It was as if the entire group had its own characteristic field around it. I also learned to see the opposite. Some people's fields would quickly shrink around certain individuals or when speaking about a sensitive topic.

Night walking began to take on more and more meaning. I was getting so good that I started trail running during the new moon. This was intense because I couldn't afford the luxury of a single thought or I'd turn an ankle or fly into the bushes. It became a powerful meditation tool and forced me to be aware and awake because my life actually depended on it much of the time.

I share this story because talking about energy fields is interesting, but it is nothing but talk until you experience them yourself. I was way too intellectual and in my head about this until I actually learned to see it for myself. The occasional flash here and there could be attributed to many things, but being able to do it on call was what really rounded out my knowledge of the matter. It became an experience instead of a belief.

The Big Picture

The truth is that we are beautiful beings of light who are all part of an ever-growing fractal called life. A fractal is generally "a rough or fragmented geometric shape that can be split into parts, each of which is (at least approximately) a reduced-size copy of the whole."[5] Apparently, any small piece of the universe has encoded within it the image or signature of the entirety—just like a hologram or our DNA. Thus, everything that we do helps create and further all of Creation. It is all beautiful as it is ever revealing itself to us. It grows around us and mirrors our internal state and mental images back to us. There is no outside versus inside, as we are all One—we are all part of the same fractal, with each part being an exact replica of the whole.

So, you may ask, shouldn't we be feeling better? Well, yes, but not in the way you may be thinking. Feeling better requires us to exist in a state of letting go, not in a state of feeling desperately bad and trapped and longing to feel bliss. It is also not a state of poverty, praying for wealth. It is a state of letting go and observing, of natural unfolding and healing. The governing principle of this universe, as discussed earlier, is chaos, which is always chipping away at the sanctity and integrity of our energy field, driving us toward death and annihilation. Chaos drives our thoughts to density and allows us to slowly sink into sleep and oblivion—only to be reborn each day to try the lesson again. It becomes a sort of gravity pulling us down into sleep. It is what feeds off the energies trapped in our shadows, and it is what supports the internal "demons" we have created.

As Leonard Orr so aptly put it, many of us are living with a pre-programmed "death urge," which drives our belief systems to take on aging and disease when we believe it is time. This death urge is both personal and societal, and at this point, it sometimes seems the United States is in a race to the bottom on the international stage.[6]

Sounds terrible! "Is this my awful fate?" you ask. *Only with ignorance and a lot of effort toward sustained ignorance would it be.*

But before you think sustained ignorance is a foregone conclusion, remember this—the energy of life is moving toward *more* life and the enhancement of itself. The key is to enter your natural state and allow life to work through you. Life is moving toward *evolution*. It is driving living systems to grow and become more and more self-aware, away from ignorance. The balance point of gravity is what I like to call *levity*—the upward-cleansing movement of integration and transformation. We are to take the "lead" of our daily experience and integrate it back into our lives to make "gold." This is the true secret of inner alchemy. It is the reconciliation of past memories and emotions back into the free flow of our energy field. It is a release, and there is no effort required in releasing. As a matter of fact, all of our effort and energy is constantly going into holding on *so we can release and become whole*. As we do so, we forgive our past and heal our wounds. We allow our energy to flow and allow ourselves to evolve and literally "turn on" our energy field.

The energy of all Creation is surging through us at all times; we are the ones who put our own energy into trying to stop this flow because we are not okay with how we feel. Once the Light Body is activated, however, the self-perpetuating light from within eternally sustains our energy field, and we are complete, never to collapse under the weight of chaos again. (Later chapters explain the process of igniting the Light Body.)

As the ancient Egyptian mystery schools explained, when we are enlightened, we are born a "star" and have completed our task in the Earth school. We become a source of light unto ourselves and, once "ignited," become a beacon for the further transformation and evolution of our species. Once we attain this enlightened point, we no longer need external sources of energy or information, as we have become One with Source and are actually an emanating focal point for that one energy.

There is something that stands between us and our natural state of divinely guided consciousness, though—the nature of our suffering and the way we leak our energy into the shadows of our unconscious behavior. We need to examine and understand this mechanism so we can learn how to unravel our problems. Once we understand the mechanics of this system, we can be fully empowered to change the way we operate, and with this, we can become free. The next chapter is devoted to this understanding.

2

THE NATURE OF SUFFERING

Now when you turn the light around to shine inward, [the mind] is not aroused by things; negative energy then stops, and the flower of light radiates a concentrated glow, which is pure positive energy.

LÜ TUNG PIN, *The Secret of the Golden Flower* (translated by Thomas Cleary)

The only way to understand a given solution is to fully examine the fundamental problem and address it. If our pure undifferentiated state is one of infinite energy and connection with the Divine Universe (call it what you may; I use various conventions throughout this work because there is only One), then our *essential nature* is perfect as it is. *Therefore, we are doing something that is causing all these problems.*

This is where the contribution of the Buddha comes in. Gautama Siddhartha Buddha lived from circa 563 BCE to 483 BCE. He was born into an aristocratic family and knew nothing of poverty and distress until one day, when he looked upon his subjects and observed things that shattered his paradigm. He could not reconcile in his mind the pain and suffering he saw in the people of the kingdom with the comfortable life he had been led to believe was the norm. This experience forced him to leave his princely life and travel throughout the countryside, looking for the answers to the meaning of life and the nature of suffering. Fortunately for us all, he actually figured it out. As the story goes, he sat under a Bodhi tree and decided not to get up until he had discovered the truth . . . which finally came to him. *He woke up.*

When people around him saw the transformation this awakening had visited upon the young man, they pleaded with him for an explanation—a way out of their own suffering. They could see that they were asleep and that this man was awake; they languished in night, and he lived fully in day.

I will not go into a full study of the nature of Buddhism here, but I will circle in on the major points we are going to examine in this chapter—namely, life is filled with suffering that is caused by our ignorance. This ignorance is what separates the sleeping from the awakened. It is an ignorance of the essential nature of our mind and how things come to pass.

The core teaching of the Buddha is that when we become attached to the thoughts that are running through our mind, we create attachments in the form of either aversions ("I don't like that; please make it go away!") or cravings ("Ooh, that's wonderful give me more, more, more!"). Once we bite, we've created a cycle of suffering. This is what one of my meditation instructors, Master Yo Hoon, calls the Bermuda Triangle, alluding to the famous region in the Caribbean where ships and planes have historically gotten lost or trapped. This is what I call the Triangle of Aversion.

For example, Judy at work makes a comment you don't like, and you think, *Wow, that Judy really is a piece of work! I wish she'd get out of here. She's ruining my lunch break.* You have created an aversion to Judy and her presence. Actually, you have an aversion to the whole idea of her. So instead of just letting it pass, every second she's there, you can't help but focus on what's wrong with her. *Why is she still talking? Maybe I should comment on those ridiculous shoes she's wearing. Does anybody else think so? I mean, really—look at how she used three napkins.* And so on and so on. Next thing you know—*poof!*—there went your entire lunch break. You spent it in your head, being pissed at a lady who was just having a rough day and had no intention of upsetting you. Or maybe she did. Who cares? But the next time you see her at lunch, all the same thought trains pull right back into the station of your mind. This time you're convinced that she's worthless, and you make sure she notices you putting your stuff in the spot beside you so that she can't sit there. That'll show her!

Maybe her dad died that day. Maybe she was coming down with a cold. Maybe she was bitter at the world for no good reason at all. It doesn't matter. You are responsible for your own reaction to an event, because *it is not the circumstance that causes the suffering but your reaction to it.*

Figure 2.1 shows the Aversion Triangle: you (the one actually suffering), Judy (the current perpetrator), and your strong desire to not have her around (the polarity switch). This is a vicious cycle.

Let's look at another example. This time Judy is someone deemed likable in your mind's eye. She always says the sweetest things and makes you feel better about yourself. Today, you've had a rough sales meeting because something you forgot to do caused a huge problem over in the fulfillment department. You need a hug, and Judy is usually your gal. Unfortunately, unbeknownst to you, her stomach is aching, and she can't see past her own pain to be showering anybody with anything today. You nestle up next to her, make some pleasantries, and wait for your Judy fix. It doesn't come.

You can't believe this! Even Judy thinks you stink. The one person who has always been in your corner is now ignoring you. How could she? So you keep fishing and fishing, trying to get Judy to renew her love for you. You want her to make you feel the way she always does.

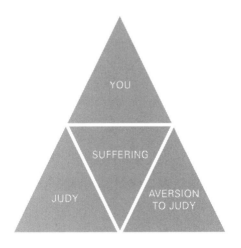

FIGURE 2.1   The Aversion Triangle

This time the triangle looks like figure 2.2: you (notice how you're always involved in all your problems), Judy's love (which you crave), and *more* of Judy's love (which she just hasn't released yet). Again, you've jumped outside of yourself and are hopelessly straining to change the outer universe to serve your inner needs. You're stuck within the tight geometry of a Cravings Triangle, which, in this case, is the confines of the scenario with Judy.

This is where our energy goes all day, every day. This is the nature of suffering. We incessantly try to bend reality to our will because we are not okay with how it presents itself to us. This, my dear friends, is the birth of impedance, the blockage of vital force in our energy field. We misdirect all our energy into trying to "fix" reality to fit our demands of it. When it refuses to bend to our will, we feel things we don't want and must force ourselves to "move" to the opposite feeling in an attempt to run away from failure. This issue warrants an example because it is an important concept that we will deal with again in this book.

Let's say you get dumped by your girlfriend in high school, and the experience is terrible. You, at the wise age of seventeen, were sure that you had it all figured out and that you were going to marry this girl. But she decided differently, and you are now crushed. You feel

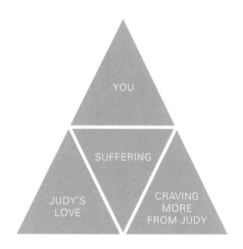

FIGURE 2.2   The Cravings Triangle

abandoned, detested, unworthy, weak, insignificant, and hopeless. Sound about right? So, how long do you stay with those feelings?

The truthful (usual) answer is, "As little as possible"! You do whatever you can to get your mind off that pain and move on. You drink, you play hours of basketball, you shave your head, you go out with the girl from your history class. You do everything short of cutting off your head to avoid feeling so miserable. Right? Or maybe you do the opposite. Maybe you start to identify with the misery and crave more of the attention it brings you. Maybe Mom feels sorry for you and lets you stay in your room and mope with no more chores for a while.

So here's the problem: those initial feelings and emotions get stored in a data bank and never go away; nothing ever goes away. The intense charge around those stored emotions is the problem. We tie ourselves down every day when we put away emotions, which then go unobserved and unresolved. Every time we have an aversion to or a craving for a particular subject and keep putting energy into it, we create a charge that doesn't go away until we release it. We enslave ourselves with little power cells of emotional baggage that eventually whittle away our energy field and our ability to live fully in the present.

Think about the original scenario this way: you were dumped by the high school girlfriend, and what happened? Because you didn't like the way you felt, you put a tremendous amount of energy into the *opposite* feelings of joy, happiness, and feeling desirable, which, at the time, made you feel like you were pulling out of that mess. Instead, *you created a monster*. See, there is the energy of the traumatic event and then the opposite energy you created and infused into that emotional field every time it came up. As you averted the traumatic energy, you created polarity. You created a positive and a negative pole for this issue, effectively giving it a life or energy field of its own. Because the same lesson comes up repeatedly in different flavors throughout life (the next girl, your business partner, etc.), you continue to charge the original aversion with more and more energy. Now it is part of you. It lives in the shadow of your energy field (because it is unconscious) and feeds off your vitality. It has actually begun to restructure your personality. Maybe you're now bipolar, or maybe you hate women deep down inside but fancy yourself as a playboy who just hasn't found someone who is loyal yet. All of this stems from aversions and craving. We move to the opposite of what we feel and create a cycle of suffering.

For those of you who are wondering how this works with cravings, it's simple: there is what you *have*, and then there is *more*. What you have is here, and what you want is there. You put energy into the future of *more* and create a gap between what you have now, which is unacceptable because you may lose it, to what you must have in the future to make you feel safe about never being without it. Like money—what if it runs out? You may think, "I need to stockpile all I can because I remember being broke, and that really sucked, so I can't have that. Therefore, I need to sell more cars this month, I need higher quotas, I need more clients." Don't get me wrong here. There's nothing wrong with making a living—a really good living at that—but be mindful of the underlying energy driving your action. Is it right livelihood? Are you running from your past, or are you blissfully contributing to society?

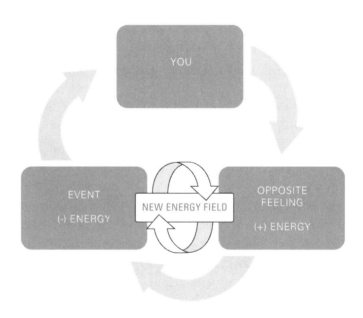

FIGURE 2.3   How Suffering Creates Trapped Energy

It's all a game of Ping-Pong in a way. We feel a certain way, and we say to ourselves, "Wow, that really feels terrible." So we volley by running out to a movie or calling that friend who always comforts us. By volleying, we start to create the spin—the other pole for a negative emotional energy field to be created, as shown in figure 2.3. Then another event in life happens that triggers the same, so we run back to our safe ground on the other side (volley with some margaritas at the beach this time). It happens again and again until we have supercharged an energy field around this sucker that can power three city blocks. It all lives under the radar of our awareness and, thus, silently drains us of our vital life energy, leaving holes in our field for chaos and entropy to set in. It makes us suffer and age, and all the while we're thinking that we're doing everything we can to live a better life and be happy.

Is this starting to make sense? I hope so, because you're going to have to understand this mechanism first before being able to rectify the situation. Then, you can start cleaning your way to freedom and clarity.

PERSONAL JOURNEYS   The Chicken Is the Buddha

I was in Lima, Peru. It was 1998, and I had taken a couple of months off to travel in the ancient Inca lands. I had always been fascinated by Machu Picchu and was determined to spend some quality time there.

I had decided to see the countryside by traveling from Lima to Cusco by bus. I wanted to travel as the locals did and have some exposure to the culture. It was a thirty-hour bus ride in the most uncomfortable seat I had ever been in. We had a number of mechanical problems with the bus and were delayed for several hours. The driver made occasional restroom stops right off the road. I remember waking up from a nap to the squirting sound of diarrhea just outside the bus; one of the passengers was squatting just ten feet away from my window, relieving himself in a nonchalant public display. Nobody else seemed to care.

After taking care of my own business, we got back onto the dirt road and kept driving into the night. The windows were down, and cold air, mixed with dust from the road, kept blowing in. I sat between two rather chubby local women who had both fallen asleep. Each had her head on one of my shoulders. The bus was loud and cold, and the rattling seat was jamming into my tailbone.

We had another ten hours or so to go, and it was only 2:00 a.m., which meant it wasn't going to warm up any time soon. I was *miserable*. As I sat there, tumbling down chains of negative thoughts, I was suddenly shocked back into the moment when someone's chicken, which had been clucking around the bus, jumped up onto my head and just sat there!

That's when it happened. I snapped out of it. I was finally able to step outside of my story line and get a look at how incredibly funny the whole thing really was. Both my arms were pinned by the sleeping Peruvian ladies, and there was a chicken hanging out on my head! The thought of how ridiculous I must have looked took over, and I started to laugh to myself. In that moment, all my self-pity and mental noise just went away simply by my developing a new angle on the story. It was not miserable anymore—just incredibly funny. If only my friends could see me now! Sometimes the power of perspective has to jump right up onto our head for us to wake up I guess.

The Cup

Here's an example that may help you wrap your mind around the concept of suffering. Imagine being a teacup. You are a ceramic cup designed to hold whatever liquid comes your way. You are filled one day with tea, another with coffee, and another with lemonade. Maybe some wine or some cod liver oil comes through the next day. Whatever it is, you then get rinsed and dried and are ready to bear whatever comes along the next day. No problem, right?

Our problem as humans is that one day tea comes in and we say, "Tea? Why would they give me tea? They know I like coffee!" Or maybe they pour coffee and we think, "I love this particular coffee. I hope they use it again tomorrow. Oh, God, please make it be coffee again tomorrow!" On and on we go, worrying about the contents of the cup, not realizing that the contents are transient. We are the cup, and we can hold whatever comes our way; when the liquid is gone, we are still the same cup. Without the rollercoaster ride of anticipation, worry, and grief over the contents, we can simply be a cup and embrace whatever passes through us, knowing that what may come will eventually move through. There is no need to hang on, no need to struggle and wish for better days, and absolutely no reason to budge reality. The mind works exactly in this way. One thought will come in and literally "bump" the previous thought out, on and on and on eternally. If we don't bite and jump in with our emotional reactions, however, the mind can be left to its own devices, and we can passively observe and be.

Some would say, "Well, that sounds pretty boring. What you're saying would mean we all sit around like useless blobs all day and do nothing." That's not the case at all.

We have all been born as little holographic flames of the One flame, and the energy of life is naturally moving through us and naturally driving us to the fulfillment of our personal dreams and destinies. Plenty of inspired movement comes from being present and tranquil. But in our modern society, we have somehow equated the lack of chaotic strife and incessant noise with a lack of drive and initiative. Get out of your own way and see what drive really is. It comes from within, and it is effortless.

The Law of Karma

Karma is action, and action is karma. We hear this word, *karma*, used all the time nowadays (often incorrectly); many people associate it only with past deeds and some kind of good deeds score to be constantly tallied up throughout life. Well, all action is karma that is either in harmony with Creation or not. It either perpetuates order or feeds chaos. By now, the mechanism should be becoming clear to you.

If you struggle against feeling a certain way and bolster your intent into an opposite energy, you create polarity, imbalance, and negative karma. This means you create more work to do at a later date. This is work that needs to be worked off or karma that needs to be cleared. You are not living in the present moment; you have socked away a lesson for later by encapsulating it in *time*. You have created a polar charge around a particular issue, thought, or memory. You tell yourself, "I can't deal with this right now, so I'm going to put it away for later when I am stronger, richer, better looking, have more energy . . . ." But, you see, tomorrow brings its own set of crap you can't handle, and that means you will never have time to deal with the issue you just tucked away. You just keep putting things away every day, charging them and filing them for a later date.

It's no wonder that many of us complain about fatigue by the time we hit our thirties. We are filled to the gills with yesterday's refuse, and yet we keep shoveling it on. There is no amount of running or push-ups I know of that can make this go away. Doing so simply sedates us by raising endorphins and allowing us to feel okay *for now*. The law of karma is not some esoteric principle outside of ourselves; we are intimately involved with it daily. All that we do creates it.

I have just spoken briefly of the chaotic side of karma, but what about positive karma? How do we create that? Simple. First and foremost is to learn to be. Sit in your heart and be the cup. Most of us think we're making a great contribution to the world by performing loving, charitable acts as often as we can, and there is nothing wrong with this. It's a wonderful thing and much needed. But ask yourself this: "Why am I doing it? Is it because God asks me to? Does it make me feel better about myself?" Maybe you're doing it because you cheated all those investors out of their retirement by making a bad deal, and you feel guilty. Or maybe you grew up poor, became a success, and now want to give back.

The point is to come from a place of balance. Get out of the cycle of aversions and cravings. Don't make the charity one side of another Ping-Pong match. Relax into your natural state and let the Tao work through you. Then, all acts are charitable, as the grace of the Divine does the work, and you don't get in the way.

The law of karma holds you accountable for your actions. Release your incessant struggle with the noise of your mind and allow things to come and go naturally. Once you get the hang of this, you'll quickly learn that most of your energy and effort has gone into this wasteful chaos. Most of your action or karma has come from this noisy mess. The more you can step out of these vicious cycles, the more your action is inspired, and the more the Universal Force works through you so you can become an agent of grace and love.

The Lucifer Experiment

One of my teachers told a story that may or may not be true, but it has important significance in the discussion of suffering. He spoke of the Lucifer Experiment, where Lucifer, being the brightest and most talented angel of God, decides he can do it better.[1] He can create a reality within God's Creation (remember, all is One; therefore, this new reality can only be inside the Creation) that is better and more interesting. Lucifer has free will, and God isn't going to stop him. According to this story, we, as humans, are all *inside* of this Lucifer Experiment. We have the choice—either to see reality as it is and *let it be*, perfect in and of itself, or to think we can do it better than God and go it alone. There is an interesting resonance between this and the suffering described earlier. It seems that creating our "monsters" or "demons" (fields inside the shadow of our energy field) is very much like this process. The shadow, by default, is unconscious, where the light of consciousness is not shining. It is where we hide that which we cannot bear to see and inadvertently give it charge. We give it our energy until it contains more power than our conscious field. This is how I believe people are driven to rape children and participate in atrocities that make us cringe. They unknowingly feed energy into their shadows until the shadow takes on a life of its own and commands their actions. Much like Lucifer was given the right to do as he would within the Creation, we step out of the free flow of the All and isolate ourselves in the dark corners of our shadow, wherein we charge unobserved emotions and thoughts that we avert until they get the best of us.

The Buddha woke up from his slumber, and those around him took note. The first step toward reconciling this tendency is awareness, which stops the downward flow of suffering and chaos and opens the channels of healing and reintegration. Awareness opens us up to freedom and transcendence.

Trance Mentality

Milton Erickson, the psychiatrist who was the father of modern hypnotherapy, was allegedly once asked what it was like putting people into trance all the time. His (paraphrased) response was: "I do not think you understand what it is that I do at all. I spend all of my time working to pull people *out* of their trances." We are a culture of zombies, walking around more than half asleep, going through unconscious behaviors that do not serve us. Because these behaviors are unconscious, by definition, we are not aware of them. They lie in the "shadow" or in the blind spot of our conscious mind and are always running. Being in the present moment means emotional reconciliation and being honest with ourselves; because we have avoided being in the present moment for so many years, we have pumped vast amounts of energy into the opposing poles of these feelings and emotions. This acts to power up their charge and make them seem like impenetrable bubbles that we don't want to pierce. As more and more of our personal power gets siphoned into the unconsciousness of the shadow, we become less and less aware of the current moment. After years of this, the empowered energy fields in our shadows are pretty much running the show. Each of these energy fields takes on a particular behavior, habit, rationalization, or story line that serves as a defense mechanism.

Essentially, when the light of our awareness shines in the direction of a charged memory or emotion, we do one or a combination of the following:

- We feel the feeling or recall the traumatic event for an instant and quickly channel energy into the polar opposite feeling (further charging the field in our shadow). An example of this would be faking the feeling of happiness when you are sad or blue. Another is spending more money than you can afford in order to feel or look rich.

- We feel the feeling and go into a story line that helps rationalize this energy, thereby empowering a false story and doing this long enough to believe that the story is true. When we do this, we create an energy field around a lie, which acts as a buffer between us and the traumatic event. An example of this would be rationalizing being afraid to talk to an attractive woman by saying that you're too busy or that her hair is the wrong color. Another example is enslaving American Indians or African slaves and justifying the guilt by convincing yourself that you are saving them. Or maybe it is talking down to a server at a restaurant because he doesn't come from your "elevated" class in society.

- We feel the feeling and react into an activity or behavior that distracts from the original pain. This happens with people who are addicted to running or who are emotional eaters—both poles of the same refractory behavior. The people who are addicted to the "positive" behaviors are oftentimes even more entrenched because they are convinced they are fine (so long as they run twenty miles today), whereas people who are morbidly obese usually understand they have a problem but don't have the right tools to resolve it.

- We feel the feeling, forgive it, and allow it to heal, dissipating the charge that has built up around it and bringing it back into the light of awareness. Absorbing this energy back into our field is what makes us whole.

Trance is the way of our culture. TV induces trance by dropping ideas in under our radar. Politicians use trance all the time by repeating slogans and mottos that call upon our fears and then channeling this energy into their agendas. In fact, society at large seems to operate around this unspoken language of the shepherd leading the weak. The weak are leveraged by their shadows. They are unconsciously trapped, and tapping into these energies draws their willpower and resources as they sleepwalk into someone else's vision of reality.

Again—the Buddha woke up. That is the necessary first step; it is also the step that needs to continue in perpetuity. We need to keep waking up to the current moment, as our tendency right now is to quickly fall back asleep. Yesterday's awakening means nothing if we're back asleep right now. To finally snap out of our trance means to understand the mechanism that put us there and to stop participating in it. We are the only ones who can create it for ourselves, and we are the only ones who can fix ourselves—period.

Now that we understand *how* this is happening, we come to the harsh realization that we are the ones doing it. We are the ones who keep channeling power into this system, and we are the ones feeding our shadows. Once we take responsibility for the core delusion that the "outside" world is what's holding us back and causing all our problems, we can finally sit back in the driver's seat (which we never left; we were simply asleep at the wheel while our shadow was driving) and take control.

The way out is *in*. Suffering happens because of our ignorance of how things work. We spend hours every day wrestling between the poles of aversions and cravings, falling asleep and waking up disappointed with ourselves that we just did "it" again. Whether that "it" happens to be eating a whole box of donuts, goofing off on the Internet when we're supposed to be writing a paper, cheating on our spouse, or conducting some atrocity, it's all a product of the same elemental mechanism—losing awareness and being driven by shadow behavior. The same mechanism that generates this cycle of suffering is what drains away our life force and slowly drags us down into ill health and broken dreams. Like the story of Dr. Jekyll and Mr. Hyde, it is our energized shadow that does all the mischief and lands us in trouble. The sooner we stop feeding our energy into the darkness, the sooner we start to wake up and snap out of it. The sooner we snap out of it, the more power we can muster to go in and release more trapped energy and vitality. Then we can start living our lives for real. It is then that we are playing what my teacher calls "the only game in town." This becomes the game of inner alchemy—turning the "lead" of our personal experience stored in our shadows into the "gold" of liberation, understanding, and true empowerment.

With a healthy understanding of where suffering comes from, you are poised to do something about it. In the next couple of chapters, you will explore basic Taoist theory to lay the groundwork for the practices in part II of this book. It is extremely important to understand *what* it is you are doing and *why* because you need to command your entire attention on this subject matter. Be hypervigilant throughout your reading of this book (and everything else in life for that matter). Remember that it all begins and ends *inside* of you. All the trapped potential and freedom waiting to burst from within simply relies on changing your understanding of reality and how truly central you are to every one of the "random" events happening all around you.

The book now turns to the specifics of the ancient Taoist practices that were specifically designed to correct this imbalance, as taught to me by my masters. To do this correctly, though, it is important to engage in a quick primer on Taoist thinking and philosophy. We need a set of rules and a language through which to practice; the next couple of chapters serve this purpose.

3

A LIFESTYLE IN BALANCE

The Way of Heaven is to reduce the excessive and increase the insufficient.

LAO TZU, *Tao Te Ching* (translated by Thomas Cleary)

The wisdom of the ancients came from something we often take for granted—Mother Nature. The Taoist way is founded on the premise that we are all One with nature and that the careful observation of nature and her rhythmic cycles will give us clues about ourselves. In fact, because we are the embodiment of the elements of nature, harmonizing these forces inside of ourselves is a profound act of union with all of Creation. The basic Taoist principles of yin and yang speak of a universal system of complementary opposites, which mutually enhance and reinforce each other. What is up without down or left without right? These concepts need each other in order to make sense. The premise of the work in this book is based on the nature of this polarity and the way in which these opposite poles interact with each other.

We often take simple things for granted. We want more, we want it faster, and we want it now. But as soon as we get it, we're over it, and we want the next thing—and then we look forward to the weekend. In the nonstop hectic world we have created for ourselves, there is no time or place for rest, tranquility, relaxation, and quality time with loved ones. Whatever happened to lazy Sundays or simple, good, healthy living?

In the excellent book *The Power of Full Engagement*, authors Jim Loehr and Tony Schwartz outlined the need for rest and recovery as balance points for our stressful daily lives. Essentially, people are far more productive when they have allowed themselves to "power down" and fill up their batteries again. A great deal of research shows this to be essential for elite athletes, but now, the same thing has been proven true for everyone else.[1] *You must rest.*

Getting proper amounts of rest should be an obvious first part of this equation, but the second part is also worthy of note, and it has to do with stress. When Hans Selye first coined the term *stress* in 1936, he called negative stress *distress* and positive stress *eustress*. But when we refer to *stress* in our daily lexicon, it always seems to have a negative connotation, even though the concept of eustress (like euphoria, which is a positive feeling) is actually a good thing for our body and mind.[2] In fact, stress is the reason we are all here: stress on biological systems has driven life toward adaptation and evolution for billions of years. Without stress, we would be blobs of protozoa. So, why is stress getting the best of us now?

The answer is simple (says the Taoist): lack of balance. We have allowed our *distress* and our *perception* of events in our lives to have the best of us. Mental stress and physical stress are different, and there's also spiritual stress. It's important to tease these out, one by one.

Physical Stress

Physical stress comes from overtaxing our bodies while not allowing them to rest and recover adequately. This may be overexertion at the gym after thirty weeks of inactivity, or it could be pulling an all-nighter and expecting to perform well the following day at work without any repercussions. These are obvious examples. How about hunching in your office chair for eight hours per day, five days per week, fifty weeks per year for the past sixteen years? That's some real physical stress on the lower back and shoulders.

Most of us can relate to physical stress because we've all been tired or injured in some way in our lives, but what about the opposite tendency—the *lack* of physical stress in our lives, which is actually reaching epidemic proportions in our country right now? This type of physical stress we are missing out on is called *exercise*, and it is good for us.

Again, remember that everything in our lives needs balance—there is the yin and the yang of all things. Too little physical stress makes the body flaccid, weak, and unresponsive. In fact, studies show that increased weight-bearing activity helps increase the production of growth hormone in the brain and helps increase and regulate sex hormones and immune function.[3]

The body likes eustress with recovery. It likes to be pushed just hard enough and then given the tools to repair itself so that it can push just a little harder next time. This is called growth and evolution.

What are these tools that the body needs? Well, *sleep* is a key, as most of the body's growth hormone is produced in deep stage 4 sleep,[4] which is the kind of sleep we get once our mind and body have settled down after running through our daily thoughts and worries. It is the depth to which we retreat for our systems to shut down and repair. During this sleep, dead tissue is shuttled away, and new healthy tissue takes its place. The body literally renews itself at night when our conscious mind (which insists on perpetually creating recklessly) goes offline and our subconscious mind can take over and handle physiological processes.

Think of Disneyland. Thousands of happy tourists parade through there every day, making a mess and leaving it in disarray. Even with the small army of employees scavenging the park all day for trash and sorting out problems, a lot goes on once the park shuts down. This is when the night crew comes out and fixes the mess left behind from the previous day. No stone is left unturned because tomorrow, thousands of people will be coming in again, looking forward to the "perfect" experience that is Disneyland.

Now, imagine that the Disney night crew doesn't do its job one night. You show up in the morning, fresh off your flight from the Midwest, and notice a half-eaten cotton candy on the chair next to the entrance. You go in and see a smashed caramel apple on the pavement. There is trash everywhere, and all the employees look tired and agitated. What happened? Well, the night crew slacked off last night, and things are a little messy. What if the night crew decides not to come back at all? Then the day crew has to work double-time the next morning to clean up and is beat by day's end. Now, how about if management decides that the park would "get more done" or "make more money" if they simply didn't close and kept the day crew working eighteen- to twenty-two-hour shifts? Well, Disneyland wouldn't be such a happy place after a week or so, would it?

Isn't this how we treat our bodies? We beat them up incessantly all day with heavy food full of preservatives. We don't take time to rest throughout the day. And then we expect to hang in there when we meet the guys for drinks or maybe see a movie with Betsie, knowing that the alarm is going to go off at 6:00 a.m. the next morning.

Exercise works the same way. We cannot do hundreds of reps of bench presses or wear out the pedals on a stationary bike and then expect results without first letting the body recover. The growth of muscle tissue comes from provoking it and slightly tearing it during activity. The body then mends these tears when we are resting by laying stronger and denser muscle tissue in the region of the tear because, obviously, that muscle is now being expected to perform more. The body allocates resources where they are needed, but it also needs the cues (exercising specific muscle groups) and the rest to stay in harmony. Providing raw substrate in the form of food (protein) is also a critical component of this dynamic and is discussed in a bit.

When we continue to challenge and provoke our bodies in a healthy way, we continue to develop more lean body muscle mass and to improve the pumping capability of our hearts. This provides us with healthy blood flow, healthy brain function, good lymphatic drainage, and good-looking skin. In fact, the steady progression of our fitness to being more and more adaptable becomes a cue for our brains to continue to produce natural growth hormone, which is a powerful chemical that literally helps reverse the aging process.[5] It makes us strong, fit, clear, and healthy, all through a natural means of continued training.

As alluded to above, proper physical rest and recovery revolve around healthy eating habits. It is also important to find your resting metabolic rate (RMR), which can be estimated using some standardized equations or through metabolic testing. From here, you can accurately establish what your current caloric expenditures and needs are and then modify your diet based on your goals. Again, there is balance in everything. If you undereat, your metabolism slows down (goes into emergency mode) and tells your body to store fat; if you overeat, your body cannot burn the extra calories fast enough and instead stores them as fat. The key for most people is to eat every two to four hours to keep the blood sugar stable. It is also important to eat enough protein with each meal or snack.

A side note: I will discuss diet and food choices in further detail soon, but I want to take this opportunity to highlight an aspect of the Taoist teaching style. In this book, we will circle around a number of topics, probing slightly deeper with each pass. This circular form of teaching is how I was taught by my Taoist teachers; staying with tradition, it is how I will address certain key topics throughout this work. Be patient and allow concepts to build on themselves. When everything is connected in the universe, we often find that we are talking *around* a central body of knowledge intellectually until we finally get in on a deeper level internally. The ancient Taoists understood the bridge between left and right brain functioning, and I will employ those same techniques here.

Our bodies are the most precious things we have. They are the chariots for our souls and spirits. They are the alchemical agent that we will later learn to transmute and refine. Learning to manage physical stress and strike the perfect balance between positive stress and adequate recovery is the key.

Mental Stress

Mental stress has also reached epidemic proportions in the West. Although it takes the same amount of time for the Earth to turn around the sun, it *seems* to be getting less and less every year. We are all slammed with our commitments. Indeed, most Americans have a commute to work that averages a hundred hours every year, according to the 2015 Census.[6]

We come from a species that typically walked several miles per day and took rests in the shade when it was too hot or when they were too tired. Our ancestors ate when hungry and had a high level of physical exertion daily, which kept their hearts pumping and their endorphins kicking. Stress came when the saber-toothed tiger popped into the cave and they had to scramble and hide for dear life.

So, how has it changed? Something happened along the way after our ancient ancestors finally stood up and began to develop the prefrontal cortex of the human brain. As we became self-aware, we began to develop a complex psyche that our animal counterparts don't seem to exhibit. With awareness of the self came the mental dialogue and the neuronal relays through the thalamus that associate past memories with emotions. These clusters of memories and emotions loop through and generate thoughts or reactions along these lines over and over.[7] Sound familiar?

Let's refer back to the chapter on the nature of suffering and recall that the Buddha had something to say about this subject. We have an event, and then we have our reaction to that event. We tend to either go toward the given subject (cravings) or move away from it (aversions); in both cases, we create a cycle of suffering. According to Dr. Alfred Korzybski, we create levels of abstraction from the original event, which pulls us and our mental energy further and further from the present moment.[8] All our power is here, now. As we allow ourselves to go barreling down our careless thought trains, we move further and further from the power of the present moment and further and further into a cycle of suffering and mental stress.

Again, there is positive mental stress and negative mental stress. We always tend to refer to the negative variety because we are all held in such captivity by it. But what about positive mental stress? The Buddha asserts that we should maintain a level of mental equanimity, which means staying in the space of nonjudgmental presence and simply observing phenomena as they wax and wane through our perception.

Positive mental stress comes in the form of healthy problem solving. Think back to math class. We are given a number of math *problems* to solve for homework. These are designed to teach us how to apply principles we have learned to a specific area and *deduce* an answer based on a certain set of rules or theorems. Once we figure out one math problem, other similar problems become easier to solve because we have gained familiarity with that type of problem. We are then promoted to higher levels with new problems and more complicated solution sets. We continue to refine our *problem-solving* skills and become more efficient at things.

What happens when we grow up? We are all complaining about the *problems* we have in our lives! But positive mental stress helps us learn how to take a particular circumstance and look at it rationally. This means being honest about all the factors and variables involved. Every aspect of a problem gets factored into its solution. Once we learn to challenge our brain and work through our problems, the game of life becomes fun.

Puzzles, math games, Sudoku, memory games, chess, and thought-provoking books are all forms of positive mental stress. But we must remember to take these on with an attitude of leisure. We cannot be the screaming kid who doesn't want to do math homework. Creating a healthy ritual of routinely challenging the mind helps the brain lay new neuronal connections and keeps it healthy. In fact, these types of activities are what are recommended for patients with Alzheimer's and other degenerative diseases of the brain. Exciting the brain with information and challenges leads to neuroplasticity (associated with youth and high functioning), while the opposite leads to neurodegeneration (associated with aging and loss of physical and mental function).[9]

It is important to remember that the mind is our tool. We oftentimes identify with the tool and get confused by thinking that we *are* our mind. Think of it this way: the mind is a product of the billions of calculations and perceptions going on in our brain, which also acts as a receiver or antenna for cosmic energy from the universe. All Source energy is here now, and our brain is the organic antenna that tunes us into it. Our mind is the self-conscious reflection of this endless activity streaming in and out with millions of bits of information. Like the guys sitting at the console watching all the funny green symbols streaming down in the *Matrix* movies, it is our challenge to separate and watch the rumblings of the machine—not to think we are the machine.

So, we must first stop identifying with our mind; we must learn to observe the perpetual motion and noise without reacting to it. Only through this mechanism can we be freed from negative mental stress and regain the bandwidth to perform the functions we really want. It is only through this method that we may find ourselves and lead a purpose-driven life.

Spiritual Stress

Many people in this day and age suffer from a lack of purpose that causes profound spiritual stress. Life is a beautiful thing when it carries meaning and purpose. We are all here to learn, love, and grow. Each heart has an earnest desire, and it is to be fulfilled. I'm not talking about getting that new Porsche your neighbor has; it's more like going on safari and seeing the pyramids, or learning Spanish and starting a winery in Chile, or maybe owning a small flower shop and reading Shakespeare at the local cafe. How about getting on board and helping to save the Earth so our grandchildren will have a planet to call home? Early humans began to move around and invent tools when adversity and necessity demanded it for survival. We're now getting back to that point on a global scale thanks to the reckless growth and industrialization of the past two hundred years or so. And let's not forget about global nuclear proliferation. Survival teaches meaning.

The truth is that each of us has likes and wants—things that make us happy. The problem is that many of us have strayed from those things and are "stuck" doing jobs we don't like; we are "stuck" in a life situation that is not allowing us the time, space, energy, or money to follow through with our dreams. So, what happens? We show up at a crappy job, can't wait until the next break, and make comments like, "It's only Tuesday?!" as the week crawls on. We then become the breeding ground for mental noise and this stagnation that takes over the system. "We" don't exist, so we assume that our mind must be it.

Let's look at it another way: assume your body is a computer and your mind is your operating system and software. First of all, how many windows do you have open at any given point? What about mental viruses (self-sabotaging belief systems)? When's the last time you optimized your disk? Do you have enough power or cooling fans on your hardware? How about updates to your software? All this sounds interesting, but something is missing.

WHAT ARE WE WORKING ON?

You could have the fastest supercomputer in the world, with all the best software, but if you just sit there playing Minesweeper, you will just get outdated and sluggish in performance. If you aimlessly browse the Internet for a while, you'll pick up some nasty viruses and maybe go nuts reading too many conspiracy theories . . . and all for what?

You need to have something to work on. Do you build houses or count galaxies with your "computer"? Do you manage money for households or create websites for newlyweds? The point is that unless there is a job or task at hand—a *purpose* in life—you could have the best system in the world, but it'll just rot away over time. Of course, this is assuming you've got a supercomputer.

Most of us have been treating our bodies pretty horribly, and we are running on low mental efficiency. We have hundreds of applications running subconsciously. When it comes time to focus, we have limited resources available for our conscious mind. We get tired and frustrated because our mind is less sharp and fatigues quicker.

It is usually easy to recognize when our performance is starting to slack. We get tired at our desk and want to go sneak a nap in the car, or maybe we read the same line three times on an e-mail and still feel confused about the author's meaning. Most of us are at least aware of the fact that our mental computers are running inefficiently. Perhaps we have taken it upon ourselves to enroll in a number of self-help courses or have read a bunch of books to fix this problem. But the real question again is: *Why?*

Once purpose is found in life, we can easily set our bearings, and optimizing our system becomes a small bump on the road. We have set off on a journey, and changing the oil filter is just another task to handle as we excitedly hurry to get going.

Many of you might be thinking, *Great. That sounds good . . . if I only had a purpose!* It is true that a great number of people are struggling daily with this notion of purpose. Remember this: nobody can tell you what your purpose in life is because you already know it. If it seems like it is fuzzy or unclear, learn to calm your mind and follow the principles in this book. You will find that the answer has been under your nose the whole time.

Our job is to learn about our essential nature and wake up to our true selves. Once we become fully aware of who we truly are and learn to control the vital energies of our mind/body/spirit axis, we are capable of creating the Light Body. We can literally slough off the dense vibrations of the physical body we arrived with and raise them to lighter, etheric harmonics. The more we evolve, the more activated our Light Body becomes and the more we are "a light unto ourselves"—rendering this cycle complete.

THINGS VS. EXPERIENCES

One of the basic habits that must be overcome if we are to pursue this lofty goal is detachment from the accumulation of things. *Things* include electronics, shoes, cars, bags, household decor, and whatever else we seem to fixate on. There is nothing wrong with these things intrinsically. But consider this: if we are considering buying a car, an eight-year-old Toyota Camry is an example of an excellent vehicle. Keeping one of these on the road is both fuel efficient and better for the environment because it takes a tremendous amount of resources and waste to produce a new car. Of course, you'd look cooler in the Porsche, but to whom?

It is also time for us all to do an accounting of the people we keep around us and really think about the games we play in our little circles. Let's say Joan got a new handbag and can now accessorize better with the red shoes she got from Bloomie's last week. Now you *need* one, too. This incessant drive to accumulate more objects to bolster our egos is causing an incredible amount of distress for us personally, and it is also destroying the biosphere! We cannot criticize China for creating all this pollution and for supporting tyrants in Africa when *we* are the ones buying the products they make. We are the consumers—the global pocketbooks that buy and buy and buy; China (or anyone else for that matter) is happy to produce *our* products for us.

Our kids' rooms are vomiting up useless toys, but we keep buying them new ones. We have too many pairs of shoes, but we insist on getting this new pair because they are so adorable. You may think, "I *deserve* this new car because I've worked so hard at this job and need to do something for myself." Great! If that's the case, sign your name on an eighty-four-month lease and pay the insurance and high gas prices to cruise around in that monster. But remember, it usually takes fewer than two months to get sick of any new car. Now, what can you buy to make you feel better?

Face it: we're crazy, and some genius marketers have figured out how to leverage our emotional turbulence by convincing us we need all sorts of crap. The solution: drop it and wake up! Get what you need and save your money. Only spend money on things that *mean* something to you.

We vote with our dollars. If we are going to turn this planet around, it is up to us. So, where do we go from here? Easy! Demand green ecology in every product. Demand that it be fair trade and torture free. If not, then *don't* buy it; instead, buy it from the outfit that does comply. Several excellent watchdog organizations will help you navigate these waters. I spent more than two years of my life interviewing the founders of the "conscious capitalism" movement in the making of my film *Prosperity*, and I can say without any hesitation that the future will be determined by the micro decisions we make every day. Money is a form of energy—feed only good things with it.

Our job is to collect *experiences* on this planet, not things. It is to share wonderful stories and have great laughs. We are here to discover ourselves all over again and find the majestic beauty in *being* and not *doing* all the time. We can spend our lives hoarding a bunch of useless crap, or we can spend it traveling the world and hiking through the mountains. We can listen to live concerts and sail French Polynesia while writing a book if we so desire. We can make our jobs and our companies stand for a green environment and help make the world a better place. The problem is that most people have given up on fixing the world, so they have resolved to live a life of mediocrity, whether they know it or not. *Wake up and live.*

In the past two hundred years, we have drained the world's resources and polluted the planet at an unprecedented rate. The writing is on the wall: this cannot last. Life is a moving, evolving thing. It is driving us to evolve to higher states of consciousness and rewarding positive traits. We will touch on this subject further in a bit, but the take-home message right now is that we cannot continue living this "American dream" and still have a planet left for our grandchildren. Stopping the insanity starts with each one of us. Buy local organic produce and enjoy meals with your family and friends. Spend more time in nature and see how it affects your state of mind. Things literally wake up within us once we have been out in nature for a while. We essentially start to harmonize with the vibrations of the plants and minerals. Our chaotic energy begins to calm down, and our mind starts to settle. With a calmer nervous system, the circulatory system becomes more efficient, and our general health begins to improve.

Here's a simple little exercise: Go out into nature and find yourself a river or a stream. Make sure you can hear running water—a river, stream, ocean, creek. Your job is to simply sit and listen to the water flowing until your thoughts begin to silence. When all you can hear is the water, it is time to get up. Practice this a number of times and allow the beauty and majesty of nature to cleanse and calm your energy field. What a wonderful start to this journey.

4

BASIC TAOIST THEORY

The Way gave birth to the One.
The One gave birth to the Two.
The Two gave birth to the Three.
And the Three gave birth to the ten thousand things.

LAO TZU, *Tao Te Ching* (translated by Thomas Cleary)

Taoism is the philosophy of syncing up with nature and doing that which comes naturally. It is very similar to the traditions of naturism and shamanism but with a fundamental distinction: Taoism bases its primary understanding of reality on the principle of balance between the forces of yin and yang. These complementary opposites exist in an ever-changing and ever-flowing dynamic state that constantly self-corrects and harmonizes. The ancient philosophers of China used the term *Tao* for the Supreme Ultimate or the universe as we know it. It is the All. In the beginning, there was Wu Wei, or the Great Emptiness, and from this came *yin* and *yang*.

Yin and Yang

Everything in the universe has a yin and yang component to it, and all things have a balance point. For example, there would be no meaning to "up" if the concept of "down" didn't exist. There is no "hot" without "cold" and so on. This primordial distinction not only relates to everything around us; it is also what fundamentally drives the motion *within* us. We, being an active functional aspect of nature, exemplify the same polar balancing; with sustained attention to this subject matter, we can find the Tao, or the balance point, in all things.

Essentially, there was the original state of the universe wherein all things were One. There was unity consciousness and eternal togetherness of all things—and then, BOOM! Polarization. All things all at once are now imbued with this elementary concept and this *perception* of separation. This is the mark of polarity. Now, it is critical to remember that these poles are the seemingly opposite characteristics of the *same* objects or things. This polarity gives us a dualistic view of the same phenomena. Yin and yang are constituent parts or mirror reflections of the same one, which is simply split into two, the same way a beam of light splits when hitting a prism. (This is a concept that will become very important in the ensuing chapters.) In the beginning and in the end, it is all Tao. Polarity is just the game we are playing.

Table 4.1 shows some basic examples of yin and yang to better illustrate this concept. These obvious examples will help further illustrate a point in our understanding of human nature—namely, the distinctions we make in our approach to self-growth and enlightenment. In our culture, we are either on one end or another. Either you work for Wall Street and drive the expensive car, or you wear patchouli and tour with the band. Either you are a democrat or a republican, for abortion or against it, patriotic or unpatriotic, with us or against us, and on and on. The mark of our society is that it is stained with the rigidity of dualistic thinking, and we suffer from its intolerance daily in our public discourse.

GRAY IS WHERE ALL THE GOOD STUFF HAPPENS!

Gray is the fusion of black and white and of yin and yang. It is the understanding that there is balance, communication, and interaction with all things at all times. We in the United States live in a culture that was started by a group of religious fundamentalists (the Puritans), who essentially lived in a world of black and white. They were too much to handle for their contemporaries in Europe, and so they came

TABLE 4.1   YIN AND YANG EXAMPLES

YIN	YANG
Earth	Sun
Cold	Hot
Down	Up
Matter	Energy
Female	Male
Passive	Active
Soft	Hard
Body	Spirit
Materialism	Spiritualism
Science	Religion

to the New World to (conquer and) live their way of life. Sex was evil, and women were witches. Everything was black or white, and there was judgment all around. It was neither fun nor tolerant.

We are now living in the shadow of that polarized thinking, and the national discourse echoes that imbalance. The insanity of the Red Team–Blue Team mentality has allowed us to stray from our humanity and has really watered down the quality of human intellectual interaction, the meeting of ideas, and peaceful disagreement. Fundamentalism (in all religions and creeds) is a child of this imbalance; it is a reflection of our collective ignorance—our ignorance of the truth.

To attain balance in the world outside of us, it is important to realize that we must first establish that state *within* ourselves. The external is simply a reflection of our internal state. Therefore, any balance we would like in our lives must come from a genuinely balanced state that originates from inside of us. We are the holographic projectors, and the "reality" we see beyond our flesh and blood is simply the reflection of our internal state. As the ancient alchemical axiom attributed to Hermes Trismegistus states, "As above, so below."

Yin and yang represent the totality of Creation from opposite sides of each other. Together they are whole, and together there is balance. One cannot exist without the other, and we cannot examine anything without a balanced frame of reference, which requires looking at both sides and finding the middle. The polarity created by yin and yang can be compared to (if we so dare) the breath of life in biblical texts. At first, there is only Tao in this differentiation. Then, movement begins, and the energy of life starts to stir and revolve around itself, swirling the myriad things in the universe into being. It is as if a centrifugal and centripetal force erupted simultaneously, both creating and destroying, rising and falling, growing and decaying. In balance, the universe sustains itself and grows slowly in sentience and capacity. We can compare it to an oak tree. It grows a bit every year and then sheds weak branches in the autumn, which then become mulched as compost for the tree's own growth the following season. The tree eventually grows so big that the main branches cannot support their own weight, and they collapse, only to become the soil for the seeds of its progeny to grow up strong and repeat the cycle.

The early Taoists learned everything from observing nature, deep introspection, inner energy cultivation, and development of gnosis. They discovered the principle of yin and yang to be the impetus and

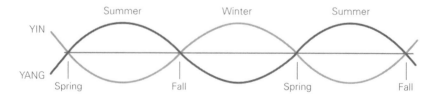

FIGURE 4.1   Yin and Yang Seasonal Interplay

driving force of all life, and this concept is inextricably linked to everything else we will discuss in this chapter.

Yin and yang can also be thought of as two inverted waves that are flowing along a central axis. In figure 4.1, we can see the interplay of the seasons and how they relate to the rising and falling tides of yin and yang. The equinox points are when the forces come together on the axis, and the solstices are at the extremes of one or the other.

If we then take this interplay and add an element of *torsion* or twisting into a three-dimensional model, we end up with something that looks the double helix of a DNA molecule, as shown in figure 4.2.

This double helix DNA serves as the information storehouse for all life on this planet, and the interplay of these strands dictates which proteins are synthesized and how we express physiologically in nature. So too, this remarkable dance between the polar forces directs the language of internal energetic communication and becomes the basis of much of our transformational work.

The Three Treasures

Once the universe is split into the polarized binary system of yin and yang, there arises a distinction between the different levels of material manifestation. If spirit and matter, which at the level of the Tao are one and the same, are separated with the birth of yin and yang, then we start to see a scale of densification versus illumination. Keep in mind that yin and yang are relative to each other, always. There is

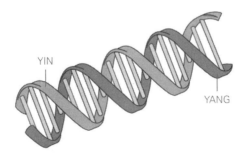

YIN

YANG

FIGURE 4.2   The Double Helix of DNA Resembles the Interplay of Yin and Yang

no absolute yin to speak of; things are only yin when *compared* with something else. We can say "hot" when it's 100 degrees out, and we could say that this is very yang, but that assumes that an average day is, say, 72 degrees. A 100-degree day would certainly be more yang in this instance. But what if we compared that to a 350-degree oven or the surface of the sun? The 100-degree day would be more yin compared to these. There is a density "gradient" from spirit to matter, as shown in figure 4.3.

Now, taking this gradient as an example, we can hold it as a frame of reference for the Taoist understanding of the Three Treasures: jing, qi, and shen. The Three Treasures also can be organized on a density gradient, as shown in figure 4.4, with jing being the most yin, or most dense, and shen being the most yang, or least dense.

The polarization of spirit and essence creates the currency of life (the qi energy). It is the medium or language of communication of All That Is. This is why it is so powerful to work with qi. When we understand the dynamics of qi flow in our body, we can begin the alchemical process of bringing the poles of spirit and essence back to a balanced equilibrium. In the duality-free stillness, we have direct access to the

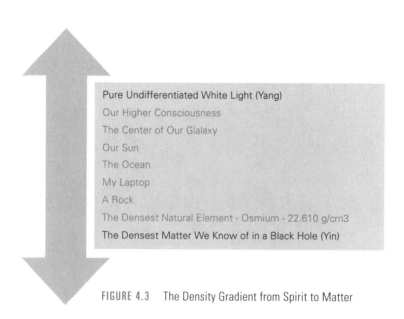

FIGURE 4.3   The Density Gradient from Spirit to Matter

zero-point energy field and are capable of rewriting the code of how we manifest in three dimensions via our DNA.

A useful example is to compare these Three Treasures to a candle, wherein the wax is the essence (jing), the flame is the energy (qi), and the aura around the flame is the spirit (shen). The goal is to preserve the essence (wax) and sustain a healthy flow of energy (flame) so that the spirit (aura) can soar. This is a very simplistic example, and much more will be said about this in part III. But before we go there, let's look at each of the Three Treasures individually.

JING: ESSENCE

Jing is the essential vitality that is stored in our body. Remember, the Taoist understanding of reality is intimately tied to the internal understanding of our body and the movement of the life force through us. To understand these dynamics is to gain enlightenment universally. Jing is the most yin of the three treasures, and it represents the core of our material existence. It is a most precious substance that is to be cherished and guarded.

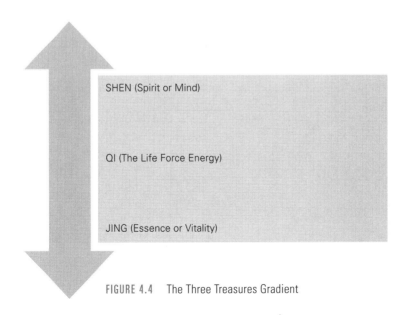

FIGURE 4.4   The Three Treasures Gradient

Very similar to the way that polarity created the spectrum of energy to matter, the essence is differentiated as well. We have our "pre-heaven" essence, our "post-heaven" essence, and our "day-to-day" essence.

Pre-Heaven Essence

The pre-heaven essence comes from the blending of the sexual energies of our biological parents. This energy nourishes the embryo and the fetus during pregnancy and essentially comes downstream from our ancestral DNA. It determines our individual, constitutional makeup, strength, and vitality and is what makes us each unique.[1] It's the hand we've been dealt by our parents. A tremendous amount of history, information, and karma comes through our bloodlines via the DNA that gets registered at this level of our essence. Microbes and gut bacteria also play a role here. Some people are blessed, and many others come in with a number of challenges in regard to this. Now, this is the aspect of the essence that's the hardest to increase, and much of the information in part II will unlock the secrets of how we can do just that through the practice of qi gong. This is an integral piece of the puzzle that must be addressed in our energetic cultivation.

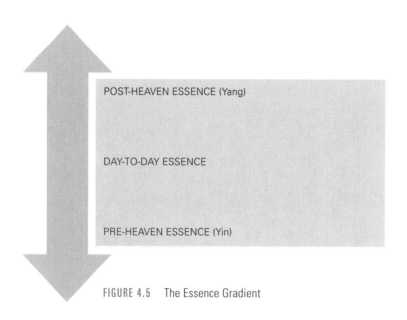

POST-HEAVEN ESSENCE (Yang)

DAY-TO-DAY ESSENCE

PRE-HEAVEN ESSENCE (Yin)

FIGURE 4.5   The Essence Gradient

Post-Heaven Essence

The post-heaven essence is attributed to our lifestyles and is quite changeable. It is what we derive from foods and fluids after birth. It's what we do with ourselves once we've come into the world. It has a lot to do with early-stage development and the quality of our nourishment from our birth onward. There is a great deal to say about this topic in regard to healthy bacterial colonies in the gut, breastfeeding, quality of foods, and the loving environment a child is brought into. A whole chapter is devoted to this in part II.

We can't really help what happened before conception or during our infantile development (though, of course, we can do so for our children), but we certainly can help what we do with it from there. This aspect of the essence really can be cultivated and positively affected by lifestyle and practice. In fact, a critical aspect of our practice is to continually refine our essence and increase the amount of condensed jing to work with.

Day-to-Day Essence

If we were to use money as a metaphor, the pre-heaven essence would be a locked-away family trust account that we know is there yet is relatively inaccessible in our day-to-day dealings. Our post-heaven essence would be our money market savings account; we can tap into it—but at a price. And then our day-to-day essence would be our checking account, being deposited to and drawn upon daily for our various needs.

Being derived from the other two types of essence, the day-to-day variety can tap into both the pre- and post-heaven reserves and replenish itself. It serves as the body's primary backup system. It acts as the reinforcement for all the body's energies, like a backup battery, supporting our systems when there is an outage. You can also think of it as the overdraft protection on your checking account. It is critical to keep this system healthy for day-to-day functioning in order to maintain health. If we want to *enhance* our health and state of being, then that is where the practices offered in this book serve their purpose. We shouldn't be just making ends meet every day; instead, we must be in a state of relative overflow and abundance. This will then give us the energy we need to cultivate strong Light Bodies and open up our perception.

So, although this form of essence is the easiest to access and can be more readily restored, it is still considered *jing* in the scale of density. It is the baseline backup system for the qi, or energy flow, of the body. Going back to our money metaphor, in relation to the other aspects of essence, our day-to-day is more liquid; *however*, in relation to our qi or energy flow, it is like a fixed savings account. Again, notice how yin and yang are always relative and how they create a spectrum for comparison. Essence is denser than energy and is therefore less "liquid" in cash flow terms. Our essence is our equity. Yes, we can borrow against it—but at a cost. The point is to store it up and create an endowment that propels us into eternity.

QI: ENERGY

Moving up in refinement from the denser essence, we have our second Treasure, which is our energy. This can be likened to all the metabolic and physiological processes in the body that are constantly running. This qi energy is the currency of life. It is always moving and in flux. It is traveling through an energetic matrix or network of channels throughout the body, called the *meridians*. The Taoist masters knew about these pathways of energy flow for thousands of years; in fact, these pathways are the basis for the practice of acupuncture.

Taking the example of the candle, the energy is the flame; it is what sets things in motion. An unlit candle can be considered potential energy, but it takes that spark of life to get things moving and really make a candle fulfill its purpose, which, in this case, would be to light up a room. Our energy works in very much the same way. It is the life force that comes into a fertilized embryo (once spirit is imbued with matter) that really gets the show on the road; that same energy carries us through our adult lives, helping to fulfill our purpose.

Now, the ancient Taoist masters spent countless hours meditating, cultivating, and studying these phenomena. From them, we have come to understand that there are several types or *qualities* of this energy to speak of.

Original Qi

This form of energy is essentially the energetic equivalent of essence. It is essence transformed into energy. Being a dynamic and rarified form of pre-heaven essence, it is essentially the foundation of all the yin and yang energies of the body. The original qi serves many purposes in the body; it is almost like a fire starter. When other forms of energy are incorporated into the system, it is this original qi that "activates" them and sets things in motion. In turn, this energy is constantly nourished and replenished by the other post-heaven sources of energy, which we are about to discuss. This original qi is housed in the "gate of vitality," between the two kidneys, and becomes a very important and active agent in our practice of qi gong.

Food Qi

As the name suggests, food qi is the energy we derive from the food we eat. This is the essential first step to having healthy energy flow in the body, and it stresses the importance of having a clean and healthy diet. This is where the stomach receives and the spleen (and the pancreas) transforms our food into a usable form of energy, which it then raises up to the lungs to mix with air.

Gathering Qi

This form of energy, which is housed in the chest, is derived from the food qi mixing with air. Once the raw ingredients from ingested food are assimilated, they need to mix with air to form gathering qi. This idea really stands as a testament to the genius of the ancient Taoists. In modern biochemistry, we know that in part of the Krebs cycle, there is an incredible symbiotic relationship with a part of our cells called *mitochondria* that creates what we call the *electron transport chain.*[2] Essentially, the mitochondria are part of an energy accelerator in our cells that allows us to use oxygen in a very dynamic process to help extract incredible amounts of energy out of simple sugars. Prior to this system, all life on this planet worked anaerobically (without the use of oxygen); the evolution of this cycle enabled eukaryotic cells (of which we mainly consist) to develop efficient energy-extraction systems. This was the beginning of the evolutionary pathway to more elaborate and complicated multicellular structures, of which we are the end result (as many would argue). Although the ancient Taoists did not speak in this language, they could literally *see* how these energetic currents moved through the human body; they developed a complicated and very accurate model to describe it.

This gathering qi serves to nourish the heart and lungs; it also flows downward to aid the kidneys. It is just as important as the energy we derive from food, and it becomes the emphasis of much of our qi gong, or energy work, which is described in part II. The cultivation of energy and healthy oxygenation of the system are intricately tied to one another.

True Qi

True qi is the form of energy that is the end product of the aforementioned processes. When the gathering qi is formed, it is activated by the original qi (which we called the *fire starter*); from this interaction, true qi results. True qi is the undifferentiated form of energy in the body that then branches off to perform the various functions required by the system. This energy takes on two forms in the body: the nutritive qi and the defensive qi.

- *Nutritive qi:* This is the type of energy that circulates internally and nourishes all the internal organs. It is closely related with the blood and, in fact, flows with the blood to bring energy to all the systems of the body. There is nothing in the body that does not interface with this form of energy, as it is the main "currency" of internal nourishment. Think of the true qi as the total revenues a country gets from taxes (food, air, water, and essence). In this example, nutritive qi would be the domestic spending on cities, bridges, infrastructure, hospitals, and so forth. It is designed to nourish the interior.

- *Defensive qi:* If the nutritive qi is the domestic spending, then this form of energy is the armed forces and border patrol. It protects the exterior from pathogenic invasion and regulates body temperature by controlling the opening and closing of pores on the skin. It is truly the gatekeeper to the body and needs to remain charged and healthy in order to keep us protected. In fact, at any given time, we are surrounded by billions of hostile microorganisms that would quickly invade and devastate our system if it were not for this form of energy. Defensive qi regulates immunity through the skin and mucous membranes and is itself regulated by the lungs, while also being supported by the essence and original qi. It sounds complicated, but it really isn't too bad.

This basic system, illustrated in figure 4.6, very adequately explains the flow of how the body's energies develop and are maintained. It also paints a picture of the complexity of the process. It is almost impossible to routinely eat terrible foods *and* successfully practice energy cultivation, because the food qi sits at the foundation of this entire process. It is also important to note that this system of interrelated

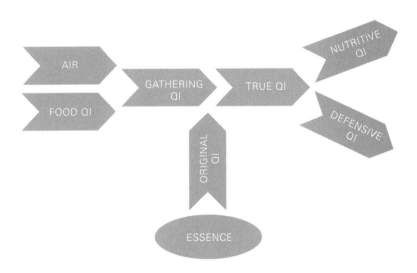

FIGURE 4.6   The Creation of Qi in the Body

energies is very much like an ecosystem that needs to be maintained. A weak defensive qi will either come from a weak true qi level or, if it has simply weakened through continual assault, will eventually drain the true qi, which backs it up at the expense of the nutritive qi.

Let's take this example on the macro scale. We have a whole host of problems in a country that can no longer pay for domestic programs (nutritive qi) because of a long expensive war (defensive qi) that is draining resources (true qi). Combine that with a faltering economy (low gathering qi) with a smaller tax base, and we suddenly get hit by both sides and have crises on our hands. Sound familiar? As above, so below.

SHEN: SPIRIT

The last of the Three Treasures is the one most people in the West are enamored by—the realm of spirit. It is the "paradise" to which we run in the West. So, it is really important to broach this subject correctly because we're walking into very polarized territory.

We live in a culture (Western Judeo-Christian-Islamic) of thinking that lives in a paradigm *outside* of the Garden. Recall that we were ejected somehow (or so says our Creation myth), and we have to behave and do as told in order to earn the rights to be allowed back into heaven—"heaven" being an off-planet realm where God and all of his angels hang out and watch us from "above." We have bought into a story line that pegs us as pathetic, materialistic sinners who are essentially wretches in need of salvation. We have to petition for divinity to intervene and "save" us from our evil human nature, which is obviously despicable.[3]

Let's *carefully* tiptoe through this mess because that is *not* how Taoists see it. Actually, there are billions of other people on this planet who see it differently, and having traveled the world a fair amount, I can say that they seem happier than us.

The Taoist concept of spirit does not exist within some far-off realm in the clouds where we'll go for some kind of afterlife reward if we behave here on Earth. On the contrary, it is right here and right now. Remember, Tao differentiated into yin and yang—therefore, matter is nothing without spirit. They are complementary, opposite *views* of the same life. When we cultivate shen (which is also translated as "mind") in our Taoist practice, we only do so by holding the critical anchor of jing and the smooth flow of qi intact. Stated another way, we cultivate the essence in the body and make it robust with life and vitality; then we use this efficiency and "excess" of energy to refine spirit further and further. This does not mean venturing into magical realms and talking to spirits as an end result; it means developing a deeper and deeper *understanding* of reality right here and now. The more we potentiate our essence and condense, the more we can *see* the universe for what it really is. Like a mighty oak tree that sends its taproots deeper and deeper into the ground, we can use these incredible bioelectric "generators" of energy that we call our bodies to literally "turn on the light" and wake up.

When the Buddha was asked what enlightenment felt like, he simply stated that he "woke up." Now, if you're reading this book, chances are you've already had a number of moments where you too "woke up." Sometimes that "awakening" is even sustained for a longer period, but the sleepy state of ignorance keeps creeping back in, like a spiritual gravity sinking us back to the lull of a sleepy zombie. In this practice, we carefully cultivate the essence and refine the spirit to *stay awake* and live in that state perpetually. This comes with an activated Light Body, which is discussed in detail later on. Our practice of taking the "lead" of our personal experience and transmuting it into the "gold" of spiritual awakening is the key to this process. This metaphor applies to the Great Work in two ways:

- It implies that we are to take our dense and powerful stores of essence and refine them into pure undifferentiated shen. This does not mean using it like a tank of gas and burning it away; instead, it connotes *fusing* it with spirit by bringing yin and yang together. We must wake up our eternal nature in every atom of our body and impregnate our material base with its spiritual counterpart so we may unlock incredible reserves of energy to wake up and shine.

- The lead-to-gold metaphor is also applied to taking the "lead" of the unresolved energies in our shadow and releasing it. It involves bringing the skeletons out of our closets and making things right in our lives. Once we release these hidden things, we'll have opened up room for the Source energy to flow freely through us again. This is the other side of the practice where we must, with our newfound energy released from our qi gong, apply the light of conscious awareness to the blind spots in our shadow.

The refinement of essence into spirit unleashes a tremendous amount of energy, which will eventually be fed into our shadow if we remain mindless. This will then rapidly highlight and magnify all the problems we are having in our lives because they will now have so much more to feed upon. Therefore, it is *critical* to practice both sides of this equation. The energy work gives us more power to apply to waking up, but only if we stay focused on doing so!

In the next section, we are going to study the concept of the five elements in Taoist thinking. These are the "flavors" through which reality emanates once movement begins with yin and yang. However, it is important to relay another fine point about the concept of shen before we do so. The five elements differentiate the shen into five aspects (remember that all material manifestations will naturally mirror a spiritual quality). The five aspects of spirit are:

- *Fire (shen):* The central notion of what we would consider spirit here in the West, fire is the house of the attention where the mind-spirit focuses its gaze. It is also the seat of compassion and love, which are the energies that intimately connect us with all life. It is housed in the heart.

- *Earth (yi):* This is the concept of the intellect—the mind and its powerful facility for concentration. It is also our ability to "digest" concepts and ideas. It is housed in the spleen.

- *Water (zhi):* This is the will or intention—the driving force of our manifestation of inner wishes and our ability to transform these desires into tangible reality. It is housed in the kidneys.

- *Wood (hun):* This is the house of the "ethereal soul," which is the aspect of our consciousness that helps reconcile the interface between the heart's desires and the physical reality that surrounds us. This is largely the aspect of us that is involved in astral travel, and it does a good deal of problem solving while we are asleep. It is housed in the liver.

- *Metal (Po):* This is the house of the "corporeal soul," which is the aspect of our soul that connects us more to the body and its lessons. Metal represents the energy of decline and the season of fall. Fall is when things return to the earth and get mulched; thus, this aspect of the soul deals with grief and letting go. It is housed in the lungs.

So, the shen or spirit, like all other things in this practice, has flavors to it. In this case, it is differentiated along the spectrum of the five elements.

The Five Elements

Once the Tao splits into yin and yang, it manifests in five distinct *flavors* of emanation that we call the five elements. The early Taoists were keen observers of their natural environment and understood that there was no separation between humans and the natural world into which they were born. The Taoists made observations about the cycles and patterns of nature, and this led to a profound understanding of medicine, agriculture, astronomy, astrology, martial arts, and philosophy. In fact, nature lies at the very core of the Taoist understanding of the universe.

Through personal connection with nature and detailed observation of the seasons and the movement of the stars through the sky, the ancient Taoists understood all reality to be represented by five elements. These elements are related to material, emotional, and spiritual matters in that they represent the entirety of our experience on our planet. But it is always important to remember that they are all aspects of the One—that pure realm of consciousness that exists in an unpolarized state. Through differential emanation, the five elements create the flavor and richness of life and how it moves and expresses itself. Remember, before the separation into yin and yang, there was the formless and unified whole—the Tao. The split into yin and yang created *movement*. With yin and yang, there are two complementary and opposing forces that dynamically flux into one another. They create the dance of life. All things move and exist through this dance, as it is the very agent of the life force itself. Now, we have further differentiated into the five elements, which give life its flavor and richness. Table 4.2 shows a basic impression of these elements, the broad range of their correspondence with the world, and how they map our experience of nature and ourselves.

We will use much of this information when we discuss how to troubleshoot problems with this framework and, more important, how to correct energetic imbalances using this system.

The five elements provide us with a greater degree of distinction on where any given thing, subject, or thought will be within its balance point of yin and yang. They show where the flow of energy is and how it is expressing at any given time, as shown in figures 4.7 and 4.8.

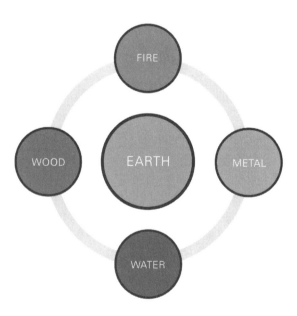

FIGURE 4.7   The Five Elements

TABLE 4.2   FIVE ELEMENT CORRESPONDENCES

ELEMENT	FIRE	EARTH	METAL	WATER	WOOD
Color	Red	Yellow	White	Blue, black	Green
Season	Summer	None	Fall	Winter	Spring
Internal Organs	Heart, small intestine	Stomach, spleen	Lungs, large intestine	Kidneys, bladder	Liver, gallbladder
Direction	South	Center	West	North	East
Emotion	Joy	Pensiveness	Sadness	Fear	Anger
Stage of Development	Growth	Transformation	Harvest	Storage	Birth
Virtues	Righteousness	Faith	Propriety	Courage	Benevolence
Planets	Mars	Saturn	Venus	Mercury	Jupiter
Sense Organ	Tongue	Mouth	Nose	Ears	Eyes
Tissues	Vessels	Muscles	Skin	Bones	Sinew, tendons
Sound	Laughing	Singing	Crying	Groaning	Shouting

In the qi gong system that we will be studying shortly, it is recommended that we stand facing the south for our practice. This explains why we diagrammatically place the fire element on top and water below. Assuming we are standing in the Earth position, facing south would put fire in front of us, with metal to our right, water behind, and wood to our left. We will use this information in the next couple of chapters when we learn how to cultivate these energies and balance them within us.

This particular representation shows the essential alignment of the elements but does not show the movement of these energies. When we introduce the principles of yin and yang to the equation, there is movement (through polarity), and we begin to see the cycles of nature manifest. We then have the four seasons.

The earth element represents the center around which all of the other elements revolve, and the seasonal elemental correspondences are closely tied to the increase and decline of energy in the annual cycle. The yang energy rises out of the winter, comes to a balance point in the spring, and is at its full expression in the summer, before it begins to decline back through the fall and eventually to the cold, quiet stillness of winter. Similarly, the yin energy picks up at the summer solstice and gains momentum through the fall. It is at its height in the winter and then slowly fades through the spring as the yang energy comes up. This entire system is simply a circular spectral

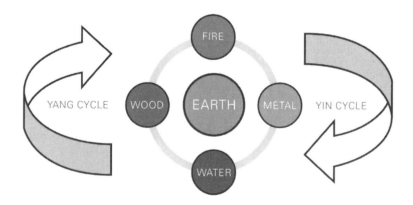

FIGURE 4.8   The Five Elements with Yin and Yang Movement

representation of the movement of yin and yang in nature. It is all the same phenomena. It has to be—there's only one reality.

Now, this system is remarkably similar to many American Indian spiritual and medicinal traditions; in fact, with proper understanding, they can be used interchangeably. Nature is nature—period. Different cultures have evolved to understand and interpret its movement in a slightly different way, but we all understand what winter is, no matter where we are from. Of course, there is less fluctuation of these seasons at the equator (where the forces of yin and yang are more balanced), and there is more abrupt change at the poles.

Figures 4.7 and 4.8 give us a relatively simple framework for understanding the five elements and their interactions with each other. They give us a reference point for our energetic practice, and they ground the entire system into something we can all relate to—nature. Now, there is another way to illustrate these correspondences that is quite useful in the realm of medicine and psychology. As shown in figure 4.9, we can overlay this elemental system on the human body, which the

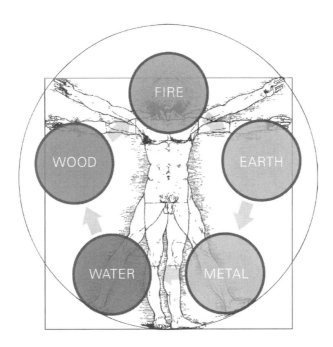

FIGURE 4.9   The Five Elements Overlaid on the Human Body

Taoists consider to be a microcosm of the entire universe, to show how these energies interact when it comes to humans.

The elements relate to each other in different ways. The generating cycle, illustrated in figure 4.10, comes from the observation and understanding that the energy of nature flows through a particular sequence in which each element is generated by another. Wood catches fire or decomposes and turns to earth, which over time settles to metal (minerals), which then returns to water (aquifer or rivers) and finally nourishes wood (plants and biomass) all over again. In this system, we call wood the "child" of water, and simultaneously, wood is the "mother" of fire.

This system allows us to understand the proper sequence of our current situation and how that relates to the overall cycle of things. For example, say we are having digestive problems (earth) due to a weak system. We can obviously help bring energy to the earth element, which is the *primary* afflicted element, but we can also put energy "upstream" into the fire element, which will then naturally flow into the earth element. Along these same lines, maybe the metal

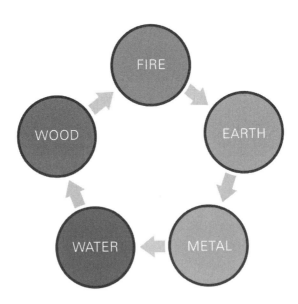

FIGURE 4.10   The Generating or Nourishing Cycle

element is what is really weak, and it's draining energy out of the earth element "downstream." In this case, we address the issue with the metal element, and the earth energy should fill back up naturally.

It is important to note that in a cycle of life, a disharmony along any point in the circle has repercussions throughout the entire system. This applies to our mind, our body, our family, and our planet. The point is that everything applies to everything in the cycle of the elements, which is why we must constantly strive to maintain balance and harmony in everything we do.

The generating cycle (also called the nourishing cycle) helps us to see the correct flow of energy through the five elements and to understand how that energy pertains to us and our circumstances. This brings us back to the concept of basic awareness in all things. To properly perceive what's going on around us, we need to look at the bigger picture and see the larger cycles of energetic movement that all things are related to. Only with this sort of bird's-eye view can we understand the nature of our circumstances and help bring harmony to energetic cycles that are oftentimes larger than us.

Using the same basic framework, there is one more relationship among the five elements that is important to understand, and that is the controlling cycle. This cycle, shown in figure 4.11, shows the "checking" or controlling functions of the elements and how they relate to each other.

In this sequence, wood controls earth, which in turn controls water, and so forth. This means that we can use a checking element to control another element that has excessive energy and is out of balance. For example, someone who is very stressed out has an overactive wood element (liver or gall bladder), which can be controlled by the metal element (lungs and large intestine). So, introducing energy into the metal organs can help control the overactive wood. This also works pathologically. Because the overactive wood element is out of control, it can easily exert a negative controlling influence on the earth element (stomach and spleen). We see this all too often in the modern world, where people who are chronically stressed out end up having digestive problems. In chronic conditions, in fact, the metal element gets drained because it's constantly trying to exert control over the overactive wood element. Because of this, we also see a decline in the metal element, which oftentimes manifests as colds and flus (lungs) or constipation or diarrhea (large intestines).

This controlling cycle is also very helpful in understanding the interplay of emotions and our mental health. For example, if a person is overcome by the emotion of fear (water element), then that element is overcontrolling the fire element (joy) and draining that system as well. We can bring in some earth energy (faith is the positive virtue) to pacify the fear and breathe energy into the corresponding organs to see a radical change in that person. That is the basis of Taoist magic. The only way to learn this and to get it right is to assume that this mystery "person" is you. All healing must originate from within. As the grand master of my tradition often tells us: "First help yourself, then help the people."

Much of our internal nei gong (or inner alchemy) involves learning how to harmonize these elemental energies within ourselves and to really use our body and mind as the workshop to figure it out and get it right. Once we learn this (and you will by the end of this book), helping

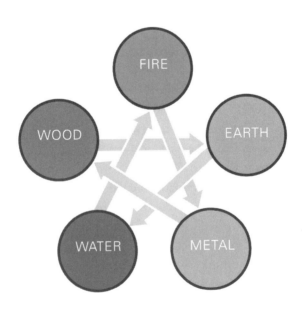

FIGURE 4.11   The Controlling Cycle

another person will be the natural extension of this skill. True, there is no separation, but most people will take that "abstract" notion and run with it. They will try to save the world without addressing their own energy first. In my experience, this is where most seekers in our modern culture fail. The central tenet of Taoist alchemy is to turn the light of awareness *inward* and to explore the universe within. From this infinity within, we are then able to unlock all the secrets of the outer world and understand our true nature. From within, we find heaven.

The Taoist way is one of peace, harmony, and honesty. It entails being aware of the cycles and currents of nature and living by those precepts. It demands that we bring the balance within ourselves to everything we encounter and to act spontaneously out of the living, breathing moment. This serves as the basic framework for our understanding of Taoism. We'll need this idea for the next few chapters, where we are going to roll up our sleeves and start tapping into our vital energy. First we'll need awareness of our energy fields, and then we'll correct the imbalances. Once clean, we will get a clear look at our true nature—which is our birthright. The path in front of us will then become quite easy, actually. Let's take the next step.

PART II

THE PRACTICE

5

TENDING TO THE PHYSICAL VEHICLE

All the faculties, possibilities, and accomplishments of shamanism,
from the simplest to the most astounding, are in the human body itself.

CARLOS CASTANEDA, *The Wheel of Time*

Our body is the temple within which we work to illuminate our understanding of reality. It is the space and time reference point where we "reside" within the fractal patterning of the universe at large. Because of the holographic nature of our universe, any part contains within it the whole. From infinity up to infinity down, it's all the same: it is all the great Tao.

Caring for our body must become the foundation of any and all "holy" practice, for our physical body is the point of view from which our consciousness experiences reality. The narrow band of the visual, auditory, and sensory information we can receive in our physical body serves as a funnel for our attention. *If we have come from an unbound universal consciousness to a rather limited spectrum of experience anchored in physicality, maybe we should pay attention to our body.* As discussed earlier, the polarized chasm in our Western thinking has created an imbalanced view of spirituality that mostly leaves the body aside, to be detested and not to be trusted. From a Taoist perspective, this cannot be further from the truth. It is vitally important to understand that the "fall" from the Garden of Eden in the Western Creation myth is not an idea shared by the naturalistic religions and philosophies of the world.

According to those traditions, we are the *caretakers* of the Garden, and our body serves as the focal point for our practice and understanding of all things.

In reclaiming the body's position as the lynchpin of our practice, it is important to address a number of vital aspects of how the body works and what it needs to thrive. In the previous chapter, we discussed the five elements and their correspondences with the organ systems of the body. This knowledge is very useful in our understanding of *how* to care for the body. In Chinese medicine, it is said that one is not to administer any acupuncture or herbs unless the basics of diet and lifestyle are first addressed.[1] That means no medicine will work if we aren't living right!

Remember, the separation of yin and yang is in our *perception*; even here, in this book, this perception has us discussing the body as something separate from our spirit. But they are all One; we are simply speaking of them separately here because of semantics. It helps us to understand the Tao when we can examine it through the full spectrum of its expression; in this case, we are examining the most physical aspect of who we are. In our practice, it all starts with the body.

The Four Wheels

In looking at what we need for our body, we can essentially break the concept of lifestyle into four categories, using a simplistic model that will help us stay focused. These four "wheels" to the vessel are diet, exercise, sleep, and mindset.

DIET

We are what we eat, and there is nothing more profound and sacred as our communing with Earth when we thankfully ingest its bounty and harvest into our body. Food is the fuel that feeds the energy of the body. As discussed earlier, this food qi is our post-heaven foundation of energy. We must eat a healthful diet filled with essential nutrients in order to have a fit and strong body. According to *Ling Shu 10*, which is one of the foundational books on Chinese medicine, the initial flow of the energy in the meridians is set in motion once nourishment enters the stomach after birth. The food we eat determines the quality and quantity of energy in our field and serves as the basis for the body's growth and development.

It is also important to note here that food holds a *powerful* place in people's blind spots. Because we have to eat so often, we often overlook our food. Food is where many people fall into a trancelike sleep, allowing the action of eating to simply fall under the radar. And while it can be difficult to bring these unconscious eating habits to light, it is also powerfully liberating. In working with thousands of patients over the past decade, I have come to understand that people who are able to wake up and actively engage in changing their eating habits are the ones who get better. It is so incredibly easy to fall into an old trance with food; almost everyone does it. To illustrate, I have been to several "spiritual" events where people are fully engaged in some truly groundbreaking work but then revert to mindless zombies during the lunch break. It often takes hours for the instructor to bring them back fully into the room. That is why most monasteries have built rituals around eating in order to keep the light of awareness on it as much as possible.

Here are a few common bad habits with food:

- *Mindless eating:* This means going into a trance or simply talking through a whole meal without paying any attention to the meal in front of us. There are often several forms of vegetable and animal life on our plate that we hypnotically scarf down without stopping to give thanks or thinking of where this food came from.

- *Overeating:* It is advisable to stop eating when just over half full. We have huge portion sizes, especially in America, and many people have walked into life with passed-down "finish your plate" mentalities. Don't waste food; simply eat less per sitting and save the rest for a snack.

- *Bad choices:* Processed foods are out. Frozen dinners are a no-no. Eat live, organic, preferably locally grown fruits and vegetables and never eat traditionally raised meats. The quality of our food is very important, and our overall health depends on it.

- *Waiting too long:* If we're starving by mealtime, it means we've waited too long. We tend to make bad food choices when our blood sugar has already crashed; physiologically, we're in panic mode. We should be eating something every two to four hours, depending on our individual constitution. This way our blood sugar stays stable, and the brain doesn't put us into stress mode. Fasting has its place, but it is not advised for the average work day.

- *Bad food combining:* Carbohydrates should never be eaten on their own. Always mix a carbohydrate with a protein or a fat. Fiber intake is about 10% of what our ancestors consumed. These help with detoxification and also feed our good bacteria.

Essentially, we want to keep our blood sugar stable and provide good-quality carbohydrates to our body. This means eating foods that are low on the glycemic index (refer to table 5.1 for a list of some "good" and "bad" carbohydrates).

Carbohydrates

Eat lots of fresh vegetables. Always start your meals with proteins and fats *first*; then, wait a few minutes before eating carbohydrates. This keeps the pancreas from spiking insulin levels in your bloodstream. An example would be dipping bread in olive oil (letting it fully soak up) and eating a little bit of that before the meal. This tempers the carb hit and gives the body lots of fat to burn instead. Ideally, however, you should dip with vegetables and avoid the bread altogether.

Essential Fatty Acids

Try to eat a teaspoon of olive oil at each meal or two or three olives per meal. This could also be replaced by a good omega-3/6 supplement formula.

TABLE 5.1   GOOD AND BAD CARBOHYDRATES

GOOD CARBOHYDRATES (those low on the glycemic index) Eat more of these foods	BAD CARBOHYDRATES (those high on the glycemic index) Try to avoid these foods
Most nonstarchy vegetables	Bananas
Apples	Breads
Asparagus	Carrots
Beans	Cereal with added sugar
Blueberries	Corn
Broccoli	Corn chips
Cabbage	Dates
Cantaloupe	Doughnuts
Celery	French fries
Citrus fruits	Fruit juices (eat the whole fruit instead)
Cucumber	Honey
Honeydew melon	Mangoes
Kiwi fruit	Mashed potatoes, instant
Leafy greens	Oatmeal, instant
Peaches	Pancakes
Peanuts	Papaya
Pears	Parsnips
Peppers	Pasta

GOOD CARBOHYDRATES Cont.	BAD CARBOHYDRATES Cont.
Plums	Potatoes
Snow peas	Pretzels
Spinach	Raisins
Tomatoes	Rice, instant
Young summer squash	Sugar
Zucchini	Waffles

Omega-3 fatty acids are essential for cellular metabolism, yet they don't lead to prostaglandin synthesis, which can lead to inflammatory response in the body (i.e., pain). You want the good stuff, and you want to avoid the partially hydrogenated oils.

Protein

- *Fish:* Eat wild fish. Hawaiian, Norwegian, and Scandinavian fish are usually not too heavily polluted. Watch out for farm-raised fish, as well as shark, swordfish, and other big-game fish, as they are usually high in pollutants. Also stay away from freshwater fish, which tend to carry more diseases and, hence, get more antibiotics.

- *Turkey:* Turkey meat is lean and high in tryptophan, an essential amino acid and precursor to serotonin, which helps feed the frontal cortex and aids in maintaining a positive attitude.

- *Chicken breast:* Poultry should be organic to avoid hormones and antibiotics.

- *Grass-fed beef:* This can be higher in omega-3 fatty acids than some fish! A healthy cow that eats natural grasses on the range is pretty healthy for you when eaten in small quantities.

- *Dairy:* Organic low-fat or no-fat cottage cheese and organic feta cheese are good sources of protein.

On top of these basic guidelines and recommendations for foods, it is important to note that in the Chinese medical system, digestion is regulated by the yang, or active, aspect of the spleen, which warms and transforms the food. Therefore, it is not advisable to eat too many raw uncooked foods, as this creates an additional burden on digestion. In fact, soups, broths, and congees are highly recommended for anyone who is having any signs of digestive insufficiency (gas, bloating, fatigue after meals, malabsorption, etc.).

Another important consideration is *water* intake. It is recommended that you drink two and a half to three liters (eighty to one hundred ounces) per day at a minimum. Spring water or microclustered water is preferable. Green tea is a wonderful antioxidant and has incredible health benefits, but it is important to not replace water consumption with this, as teas have an overall dehydrating quality by stimulating urination. Avoid coffee—it is too acidic and is also dehydrating. A great deal of research has been done on the healing properties of water, including maintaining a healthy histamine response (allergies), enabling digestive juices to be properly secreted, and detoxifying the system—and obviously many more.[2]

Drinking enough water is critical for all functions of the body, and many of us are running around in a chronically dehydrated state. As far as cultivating energy goes, things will simply not flow correctly without adequate hydration in the system.

Getting a handle on food isn't just important; it is critical! Follow the basic guidelines in this section, and you will see things begin to change almost immediately. (Please note that this text does not take the place of qualified, individualized help.) Eating well is a lifelong study, and the good news is that you have several chances to get it right every day. The take-home message of this section is one you've heard before: wake up! Be mindful of your eating habits. Pay attention to *what* you are eating and *how* you are eating it. Chew slowly and savor your food. Add more fiber via vegetables and fresh fruit. Don't talk so much while eating. Really allow the food to settle into your stomach before your next activity. Your participation in this process is not optional. This is an unconscious rug under which much has been swept. But you are the new sheriff in town. Ride in and clean up that mess because nobody else can do it for you!

PERSONAL JOURNEYS   Adjust Your Diet to Your Lifestyle

Before I found the Chinese martial arts systems, I practiced in some of the Korean arts for a number of years. After thousands of roundhouse kicks, I was starting to have a persistent achy pain that wasn't getting any better.

I was very busy with school and work at the time, so I decided to give my training a break for a number of months to allow my hip to heal. I went from thirty hours or more of aggressive training per week to almost nothing except some mild yoga. Prior to taking this break, I simply could not eat enough to keep the weight on; I probably had the ability to digest a car tire in those days. I was on fire and could eat anything.

Four months later, it occurred to me that I had forgotten to turn down the dial on my food intake; my appetite and subconscious eating patterns had been dialed into the exertion level of a serious martial artist, yet my lifestyle had shifted to that of a mellow yogi. I woke up one day having put on a good fifteen pounds! I had fallen asleep to my shifted caloric requirements and was piling too much fuel into a much less active machine.

I quickly adjusted my diet down and tuned my cardio exercise up. It didn't take too long to turn around, but it certainly wasn't as easy.

EXERCISE

Traveling through India and Asia while on sabbatical, I ran into spiritual aspirants who did nothing but sit and meditate all day. Such daily devotional work was commendable, but their bodies were falling apart because they were suffering from many of the same problems I had encountered with patients in California. The singular, shared trait was that neither population really moved. Poor immunity, low energy, achy muscles, weak joints, and low morale were just some of the health problems. The 2015–2020 dietary guidelines for Americans advise at least 150 minutes a week of moderate-intensity or seventy-five minutes a week of vigorous-intensity aerobic physical activity. They also suggest "muscle-strengthening activities that involve all major muscle groups on two or more days a week."[3]

Over the years, I have had extensive training in the Chinese martial arts, with an emphasis on the Shaolin tradition. Here's a quick story about the Shaolin temple:

In the early fifth century, an Indian monk by the name of Bodhidharma traveled to the Shaolin temple in China and took up residence outside the grounds, where he sat in silent meditation for a long time until the monks took notice of him. When invited to enter the temple to teach, Bodhidharma immediately noticed that the physical constitution of the monks was weak and sickly. He proceeded to teach them a series of mind-body exercises and introduced a more rigorous labor regimen for their day-to-day activities. With the introduction of his powerful yoga techniques (the qi gong, which we will study soon) and physical exertion, the monks began to gain strength. This heralded the start of the golden age of the Shaolin temple, wherein the monks were transformed into the famous "warrior monks." With superior skills in the martial arts, they became the defenders of good and justice in ancient China. Bodhidharma is known as the first patron saint of the *Chan* Buddhist tradition (which is called *Zen* in Japanese).[4]

The Shaolin kung fu philosophy of chopping water and fetching food, mixed with rigorous training, created a form of "superhuman," and this is nothing more than our birthright. We all have the capacity—and, I would argue, the *need*—to develop our bodies to become strong and resilient. It strengthens our bones, aids our circulation, boosts our immunity, clears our toxins, raises our metabolic rate, helps us burn fat, supports our joints, and lifts our mood. It really is a no-brainer. Yet, most people do not get enough exercise and are constantly struggling with their health and weight. Again, we come face to face with ourselves here. It is incredibly easy to come up with excuses not to exercise and to go unconscious about it, but the answer is always the same: we still need to get our exercise.

In my opinion, working out just for the sake of working out is very difficult to do, which is why most people don't do it. I much prefer sports or games. I personally train kung fu, go hiking, play basketball, or swim. Now, there's a catch to this, and anyone who has played weekend warrior long enough can attest to it: sports only work until you get injured! This is where the gym comes in; this is where functional training takes meaning. We train and increase strength in order to support the structures and to *stay* healthy enough to play sports. Sure, if you enjoy lifting weights, then you're all right. But most people hate gyms, and a majority of people in this country won't even step foot in a gym, for a variety of reasons. But, alas, we still need to move! So let's now look at some powerful ways to do so without the drama of the gym.

First of all, if you're not already taking a morning walk, start ASAP! It increases the metabolic rate for the rest of the day and cues the body to start burning fat instead of sugars preferentially. A brisk morning walk for twenty to sixty minutes, followed by a healthy breakfast, will set the energetic tone for the day and boost mood and circulation very quickly. Just build it into your daily routine. Yes, the first few days will be rough with the earlier alarm clock, but, within a week, you will likely be off to the races and will be so happy you are doing it.

Second, we *need* weight-bearing exercises to maintain good health. Weight-bearing exercise is critical for the development of muscles and bones. Basic squats, lunges, curls, dips, push-ups, pull-ups, and rows are a good way to get started—and they don't require a gym membership! What we want to do is stress (remember eustress?) the muscles into activity, which signals the brain to release more growth hormone (increasing post-heaven jing) and to further develop the system. Either we are busy growing, or we are deteriorating. We need weight-bearing exercise to support our lean muscle mass and nervous system. There is no quicker formula for aging and rapid decline than a sedentary lifestyle. Muscle development is a key factor in keeping the body-brain connection active.

Third, stretching is our friend. I would say that 90 percent of the musculoskeletal injuries I encounter in the clinic are a direct result of inadequate stretching. People are just too busy nowadays for stretching, and they really pay the price. Maybe stretching isn't active enough for you. Maybe there's no time because you just arrived at the tennis courts, and your friend is ready to start, so you pick up your racquet and strain your elbow ten minutes in. Consider stretching the yin activity for the yang aspect of your routine. They need each other.

Fourth, cardiovascular exercise is key. The legs are considered our second heart, and we need to break into a sweat daily in order to expel toxins, drain lymph, and keep the heart muscle healthy. Again, this is where a lot of people injure themselves, so it is important to stretch before and after exercising. It is also important to train the leg muscles and strengthen the lateral stabilizers of the hips in order to avoid injury when running. I'm personally a big fan of long hikes with added weight in a backpack to keep the heart rate up. Running is very rough on the joints, and most people hurt themselves trying to get into it and then are put off from exercise altogether; this is obviously not helpful.

In addition to getting the heart rate up, a little time outside communing with nature is always good—especially with fresh air and sunshine. (Note: If you have a history of heart problems or suffer from shortness of breath or dizziness, please consult your physician before jumping into a cardio program. It is always important to be safe in what we do.)

Finally, as mentioned in part I, recovery is a critical aspect to all that we do. The body needs rest in order to rebuild tissues and recover from exercise. A majority of the elite athletes I have worked with exhibit signs of adrenal fatigue, and their lab work confirms this. They are burning up their essence by pushing too hard and not allowing the yin aspect of their activity to match their drive.

Again, balance is key in everything we do. The body needs stress in order to continually evolve and grow in a healthy light. Too much stress damages the system, but not enough stress is what we have when we sit on the couch and watch the tube. Balance is the operating ideology of all Taoism, and we need to attain it in all aspects of our lives.

SLEEP

Speaking of recovery, to date, there is no better substitute for fatigue than sleep. It is an absolutely critical process that we often take for granted. It is our chance to finally lay to rest our conscious mind, which has been working so diligently all day. We have millions of bits of information going through our mind in any given second. Our conscious mind can only handle a very small fraction of that information because it has to reconcile what it sees "outside" ourselves with the artificial identity we've created (called our ego). This gives our mind a heck of a job because the ego routinely faces catastrophic collapse daily as new information challenges its definition of itself and forces reconciliation.

Now, in addition to all the energy we store subconsciously in the shadow, we also have millions of reactions to emotions we don't want to feel and memories we'd rather forget. These load up defensive arguments and chains of rationalizations, which interface with our consciousness all day. Whatever is brought into the light of conscious awareness must be dealt with by either absorbing into our greater self-identity or stuffing it away into the shadow to deal with on another day. Sleep is where much of this gets cleaned up; it's when the brain is allowed to process and make sense of the day's happenings.

Aside from the profound mental reorganization, sleep is where tissues throughout the body are repaired and toxins are expelled. Living in this modern world, we are all being exposed to toxins at an unprecedented rate, and we rely on our body's detox pathways to help clear these poisons at night. Inadequate levels of sleep severely compromise this system and force us to carry these toxins into the following day, which, as we all know, has its own load of junk to deal with.

Hibernation Saves the Day

I have read many stories about Taoist masters who really applied the philosophy of rest and recovery to their daily lives. During an extremely busy time in my life, I had gone more than a year and a half without any real down time. I was always behind on something and was constantly overcommitting left and right.

I'd been teaching a classroom full of students in Los Angeles about eating seasonally, and I was working on the next lesson's curriculum (which was about modulating our energy output to match the seasons), and that's when it finally dawned on me. I was totally exhausted and running myself into the ground. I had been so motivated to help people that I had forgotten my teacher's primary axiom: "First help yourself, then help the people." I was being a terrible Taoist.

It was late fall at the time, and winter was already showing in the trees. I had just been hit with the reality that "go with the flow" had not been part of my life for a couple of years. The "flow" should have landed me in a hammock long ago! I went about clearing my schedule in the winter and pulling my energy out of all noncritical tasks. I kept my practice and a modified exercise program.

I essentially committed to do whatever it took to rejuvenate that winter. I gave my body sleep as often as I could. At first, I'd sleep twelve to thirteen hours per night and most of the weekends. I had to *commit* to being *lazy*. I had to learn to say no to friends when the phone rang. It turned into a hibernating "staycation," and I spent a lot of down time thinking and catching up on little projects in the house. The operating motto was "rest when you're tired"—and that was pretty much all the time.

It took about three months before I really noticed what had happened to my life. The dark circles were gone from under my eyes, my achy low back was no longer bothering me, and the low-grade anxiety that had seemed to always be there was gone. It turned out that some of the mental noise had been purely physiological; it had been my body trying to tell me what it needed. In my case, I needed sleep. Eventually, I felt like doing things again and had a renewed enthusiasm that came from deep within. I was restored and felt healthy again. Lesson learned.

The next lesson, however, was soon to come. I needed to find that balance in my everyday life. Sure, I could crash in the winter after a crazy year, but that was a big swing of the pendulum. Was I going to be able to find that balance in an average day? That turned out to be the real Taoist training because it required mindfulness. I had to wake up to my daily trance trains and become an Urban Monk.

Sleep is also a critical place for tissue recovery and growth. During stage 4 sleep, the body releases growth hormone (vital essence) into the bloodstream, which helps trigger the muscles and tissues to stay young and to proliferate. This ultimate yin activity becomes the basis of our regrouping and repair at night. This is why a minimum of six to nine hours of sleep is necessary for most people.[5]

Let's go over some basic sleep hygiene rules to help you get better sleep now:

- No caffeine after 2:00 p.m. The stimulating effects can stay with you for several hours.

- No TV or other screentime in the bedroom. It sends pulses of light to your pineal gland (third eye), which signals the brain to stay awake and alert and kills your sex life/intimacy.

- No bills or stressful business in bed. The bedroom is for sleep and for making love. Keep everything else out.

- Keep the temperature cool and a window cracked for fresh air if you can. (For most people, 68–72 degrees Fahrenheit is the average temperature for inducing the best sleep.)

- No big meals three hours before bed. (However, if you suffer from insomnia, you'll want a small snack of fat and protein to stabilize your blood sugar before bedtime.)

- Write down what's on your mind so you can deal with it the next day.

It is important to note that a very healthy practice is to set out what you need to accomplish on any given day and make sure you do it before you go to bed. Don't take unfinished business to bed with you, as it'll keep your mind unsettled throughout the night. If you constantly have unfinished items on your list every night, then it is time to really look at your goals and manage your expectations of yourself. Are you being unreasonable with what you expect of yourself, or are you chatting with people at the coffee shop for too long and neglecting what you need to do? In any case, *event* management, rather than *time* management, is the key. Time is pretty consistent; it is the number of events we commit ourselves to that crunches our time and gets us stressed out. (I invite you to read my book *The Art of Stopping Time* for a hundred-day journey into this topic.)

Part of the process here is the process of becoming honest with ourselves and bringing to conscious light all the side deals. These deals are the unspoken agreements we have running in the background that cause us grief and stress. Essentially, we should choose to either drop it or handle it. Whatever it is, we need to stop dragging it around. This leads us to our fourth "wheel" of the physical body.

MINDSET

The way we see our body and the way we live our life are direct reflections of our internal state. The levels of stress we experience have a profound effect on our body. Although this book has an entire chapter devoted to Taoist mental practices, it's important to speak of this subject in relation to our body as well. The key to a happy life is to develop a peaceful "operating system." This puts us in a healthy mindset that isn't looking for a quick fix every time stress overwhelms us.

In my clinical experience, most people in the West have compromised adrenal glands because of long-term stress to their system. This is directly a result of their lifestyle practices. For example, those of us who have a hard time eating on time routinely call upon our adrenal glands to secrete cortisol as a blood sugar stabilizer. Cortisol helps pull stored sugar out of our reserves because the brain cannot go without food. As the primary organ in the body, the brain will sacrifice other systems to get what it needs. This can lead to hormonal problems, insomnia, long-term exhaustion, anxiety, and low back pain. The extra cortisol in the system tells the body to store fat (which it does when it is in emergency mode), which makes it difficult to lose weight, no matter how hard we exercise. Then, the adrenals finally exhaust our reserves, and the cortisol just isn't being produced, so the body uses the next system in line—epinephrine and norepinephrine—to get sugar. When this happens, we are jolted out of bed with a racing heart, and we have a low-grade level of anxiety that doesn't seem to go away, no matter how many trips to the Bahamas we take. Now we are in trouble.

We need to develop a mindset of reverence and goodwill toward our physical body. We must treat it like a long-abused child who now, finally, needs the extra attention and love it deserves. We need to listen to it and *ask* it what it needs and then *give it to it*. This becomes a practice of honoring the needs of our physical vehicle and raising it to its rightful place as the very altar of our spiritual practice. Remember, balance is the key.

Mindset and the Five Elements

Each of the elements is associated not only with an internal organ but also with an associated emotion (see table 5.2). Mania, worry, grief, fear, and anger are manifestations of imbalanced energy in the five elements, but they are *simultaneously* expressing as pathology in their corresponding organs. Heart palpitations, indigestion, shortness of breath, chronic exhaustion, and vertex headaches are also respectively brewing within those emotions and vice versa. As above, so below. Everything is associated with everything else in Taoist thinking, so

TABLE 5.2   FIVE ELEMENT ORGANS AND EMOTIONS

ELEMENT	FIRE	EARTH	METAL	WATER	WOOD
Yin Organ(s)	Heart, pericardium	Spleen	Lungs	Kidneys	Liver
Yang Organ(s)	Small intestine, triple burner	Stomach	Large intestine	Bladder	Gall Bladder
Emotions	Mania	Worry	Grief	Fear	Anger

physical lifestyle habits can influence mental patterns, while emotional disturbances can show up as physical ailments.

This obviously speaks volumes about the importance of caring for the body—inside and out. The good news is that the body has an amazing ability to self-regulate, so good diet, balanced exercise, and adequate sleep all go a long way in healing many illnesses, including problems with the internal organs. The point to take home here is that in order to wake up, we need to do so on *all levels*, and it starts with the body. Cleaning up the temple is the necessary first step in the alchemical process.

6

THE ANCIENT PRACTICE OF QI GONG

The breath is one's own mind; one's own mind does the breathing. Once mind stirs, then there is energy. Energy is basically an emanation of mind.

LÜ TUNG PIN, *The Secret of the Golden Flower* (translated by Thomas Cleary)

The literal translation of *qi gong* is "energy work." It is an Asian form of yoga that has been around for thousands of years. Much of it is performed while standing, though there are a number of seated sets as well. There are hundreds of systems of qi gong that have come from various lineages, and many of them focus on different fields. Many are health oriented, while a separate group comes through the martial arts lineages. These systems act to harness willpower, to focus, and to help practitioners channel their energy through their palms. There are also a number of systems from the temples and monasteries that are more focused on spiritual cultivation and depth of meditation. Some involve moving, and others are visualization based. Almost all of them involve specialized breathing, which is coordinated with the activity at hand. The guiding principle of all these practices, however, is the coordination of the eyes with the body movements, the focus of the mind, and the breath, especially for the moving practices. For the more passive, nonmovement exercises, we focus the vision inward and explore the inner realms as we guide the breath to various inner chambers.

Let's take a moment to look at this formula again to see if we can dissect it a bit more. We are looking for the coordination of all (not just a couple) of the following to take place in order for our qi gong to be effective:

- *Eyes:* In the West, the eyes are considered the gateway to the soul and, in Taoist theory, are believed to guide the shen, or the spirit. It is said that the qi (energy) follows the shen (spirit), and the blood and body fluids, in turn, then follow the qi. Therefore, the eyes become the "command center" for the spirit to control and guide the movement of the energy in the body. Later on, we will use the same system to direct energies outside of our body to effectuate healing and exert our influence on the environment around us.

- *Body movements:* These are the actual sequenced movements of the qi gong exercises. Many of these follow the pathways of the energy meridians that run through the body. They also often trace the outer edges of our energy fields, smoothing and caressing the potency of the energy flow in our Light Body. These movements often involve various degrees of exertion, and depending on the system you are training in, they can actually be quite rigorous. Recall the story of Bodhidharma and the Shaolin temple. He created a routine (called the Famous Tamo's Eighteen Hands of the Lohan) that fully mixed kung fu with qi gong with relatively high levels of exertion. This aspect is very much like the physical yoga systems in the Indian traditions. Some hold static postures, while others emphasize more dynamic flow and continuity of motion.

- *Mental focus:* This is a critical aspect of the practice and is the one that students most often overlook. Paying attention is a critical component to any energy work, as it engages the fire energy of the heart and ties the spirit in with the actions at hand. The ancients say the linking of attention and intention creates mastery in life. Here, we are asked to focus on the action at hand and to stay engaged in the body movements, tracking them with the eyes. Doing so demands our mental focus and presence, and the reward is immense. This aspect also draws on the *yi*, or shen, of the earth element.

- *Breath:* It is the vital breath that is said to circulate through the various meridians, and it is the energy from the air, if you recall, that mixes with the food qi to create the functional energy of our body. The coordination of breath with body movements and attention drives energy through the designated pathways and opens blockages. We use breath not only to open these pathways but also to gather and store the breath and energy in specific reservoirs (called dantiens) in the body. An adept student learns to extract vital energy from the air through breathwork.

As simple as it seems, it is this framework that sets the precedent for all the magic to occur in qi gong. Now, there is much to be said about the specific movements and the deep understanding of the energy pathways and how they affect us, but even if we were just to take this level of focus and coordinated thought and breathing into our day-to-day lives, we'd be far ahead of the game. The good news is that we are about to learn about these pathways, and we are going to unlock and *understand* the mechanisms of action here. We will engage the intellect (yi) and the attention (shen) with the intention (zhi). Once this "vertical axis" of fire-earth-water has been activated, we'll have finally unlocked the first hints of our tremendous potential, and a number of powerful changes will start to happen.

This vertical axis gives us the mental and spiritual alignment we need in order to connect all aspects of our being into our body while in our practice. The connection of all the various aspects of ourselves through the practice really begins to snap us out of our trances. Once we correct the flow of energy and divert it away from all the wasteful patterns of our past, we can start to gather and accumulate power in our reservoir and use this as a buffer against disease, fatigue, or simply falling back into a sleepy trance. When we speak of accumulating power or storing energy, we are speaking of creating places where we *condense* and *refine* the quality of the energy that is moving through us. We condense it to *nourish* our essence, and we refine it to *illuminate* our spirit. However, we want to be careful to not think of it in capitalistic terms. This is critical in our understanding of qi gong—or life, for that matter.

There is actually no need for *more* energy at all because there is an infinite amount of energy available to us right here and right now. In fact, all the power that ever was or ever will be is here and now. So, it is important to not get into the "acquisition" game of energy and to instead realize where it comes from. There is no outside source from which we draw energy, like water from a well. The entire force of the universe is flowing *through* us at all times and in all places. Therefore, it is the *impedance* or the blockages we create to the free flow of this energy that makes us feel a sense of lack. We channel much of this energy subconsciously to our shadow, and we simply close our minds to the limitless flow of it because it would simply break our ego's definition of ourselves. We keep our foot on the brake and then wonder why we're exhausted all the time.

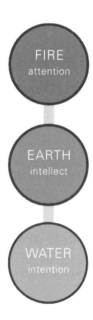

FIGURE 6.1   The Vertical Spirit Axis Linking Attention and Intention with Intellect

The goal of qi gong isn't an addition process; it is more a subtraction process. The more we can get out of our own way, the more we can let the universal flow of energy move through us. We become an agent of its goodwill, and we take our rightful place in eternity. This is not in some far-off heaven but here and now. Qi gong helps us wake up to the living, breathing moment in which we can finally take part. An important aspect in "getting out of the way" is reconciling the stuck energies in the "horizontal axis" of grief, anger, and frustration.

This horizontal soul axis of emotions is intimately involved in the rising and falling trends of our mental and emotional upheavals. It is simultaneously tied to the cycle of life and all the trials and tribulations of the soul. It is important to not be deferential about this and to be engaged in the process of reconciling imbalances on this axis. It is at this point in the process that most people get stuck because this is where they store the majority of the repressed charge in their shadows. Our desires for addition (wood) and our reluctance to let go (metal) lead to a great deal of clinging and suffering. In playing this game, we get out of balance and unconsciously pour more and more energy into creating "monsters" here.

In Chinese medicine, the lungs represent the metal element, which *descends* energy naturally, while the liver represents the wood energy, which naturally *rises*. The lungs sit *above* the liver in our body, and it is the dynamic tension of trying to maintain this inverted energetic flow that is the essence of life. One pushes up from underneath as the other pushes down. Upon death, the shen of the liver, the *hun*, ascends to heaven, and the shen of the lungs, the *po*, descends into the earth. We need them to check each other in dynamic tension; otherwise, they will separate, and we will perish.

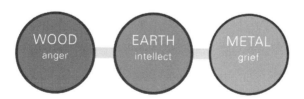

FIGURE 6.2   The Horizontal Soul Axis of Human Emotions

Bringing harmony to the proper flow of the horizontal axis is what keeps our lives running smoothly and plugs us into the power of the vertical axis. The proper alignment of attention and intention requires a healthy understanding of the human condition; far from running from it, we are to be engaged, aware, and awake moment by moment.

The Dantiens

Much like the Indian system of chakras that represent different aspects of the light as it expresses through our physical body (see figure 1.2), the Taoist system uses three main energy reservoirs, called the *dantiens* (see figure 6.3). There is a lower dantien, which is located approximately three inches below the navel between the front of the torso and the spine; a middle dantien, which is centered in the sternum (at the center of the chest and level with the heart); and an upper dantien, which is housed slightly above eye level in the forehead (the third eye). The lower and middle dantiens range in size but can be approximately the size of a small bowling ball, whereas the size of the upper dantien depends on the level of attainment of the individual—usually anywhere from a golf ball to a tennis ball in most people.

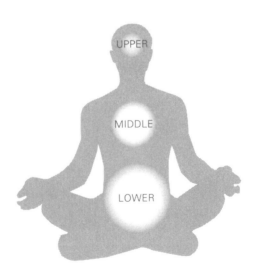

FIGURE 6.3   The Dantiens

The lower dantien is the area where we first learn to direct our breath. It is the foundation of the energy body system. The Taoists believe that it is important to start with the heaviest and densest forms of energy in our cultivation and to work up from there. Again, yin and yang have differentiated, and the heavier and more yin aspects are located lower in the body. In fact, hui yin, which is the first point of the conception vessel (energy meridian), is located in the perineum and is considered to be the most yin aspect of our anatomy. It is the base of our torso's energy field and is the point from which the lower dantien energy emerges and returns to. Anchoring the breath and the shen (which is more yang in nature) down to this region brings the first level of balance to our system. Think of it like a construction job; a solid foundation *below* gives us a steady structure above. As above . . .

What we want to do in qi gong is systematically go through and balance the energies of our body from base to crown and only move forward once we have done so successfully. We want to concentrate our energy into the lower dantien and then allow ourselves to draw upon this "core" region for every movement. We want all the body's energy currents to run through here in order to nourish the original qi and post-heaven essence. The more energy we can release to these systems, the more efficiently we can metabolize foods and run our day-to-day processes. The more we do this, the more trapped or blocked energies we'll be able to free and the more positive energy, in turn, we'll have to work with every day of our lives.

As we optimize the flow of clean energy through our energy fields, we will be faced with blockages that carry with them mental and emotional content that is deemed "undesirable"—things we've stuffed into our shadow. The more light and awareness we bring, the more our shadows will become illuminated, which leaves less space and power available to hidden subconscious processes. This can be a bit unsettling to face, but remember that we now have increased energy and awareness to deal with what's there. This is where the middle dantien comes into play. We use the energy of the heart to forgive these events and memories. We learn to disengage from our typical response of empowering these blockages by running and pumping energy into a polarized "solution." We use the lower dantien to bring up the power (almost like activating a battery and plugging into it); then we use the middle dan-tien to transform what's been trapped in our shadows, which we now finally have the strength and ability to deal with. From here, the new energy is released and refined in the upper dantien, where it becomes pure, undifferentiated light of awareness.

The more self-aware we become, the easier this process gets. Alchemy is actually quite fun once the "engine" gets going. There's always some-thing to clean—always energy to access and things to unlock. Once you get this, there will never be a dull moment in life.

PERSONAL JOURNEYS   Falling Up a Hill

I was scheduled to climb a mountain that was over 20,000 feet tall in Bolivia. I had made friends with a couple of hard-core Swiss guys in the jungle, and we had agreed to climb Huayna Potosí together. It wasn't K2 or anything, but it was pretty hectic nonetheless. We hired a guide and rented all the necessary equipment. We hurriedly got our affairs in order and were as far as the car would take us by evening. We had to hike for hours to the glacier, which was at 18,000 feet. This was where we were to practice using our ropes and ice picks for the following day. It was hard to breathe, and we spent a couple hours practicing climbing up and down ice walls that were quite tall. We then set up our tents and camped on the glacier that night.

I was having a hard time getting enough air and could not get warm for the life of me. I basically shook all night in my crappy rental sleeping bag until the guide summoned us at 1:00 a.m. We were to hike with headlamps and were to summit just after sunrise. I was happy to get going—anything to warm me up! We had some tea and some eggs and were on our way up the glacier.

Our guide was in front, with the three of us in tow behind, each a safe distance apart on a rope. It was really slow going to begin with, and it just got harder. I remember being able to take a number of steps per breath at first. As we got closer to the top, I was essentially taking one breath per step. One of my Swiss counterparts was vomiting and had a splitting headache, while the other was delusional and talking to himself. I had a mild headache and recalled reading that we were supposed to descend if we had signs of altitude sickness.

No way! The machismo spirit won out, and we decided to pummel on. I got to the point where I was taking a number of breaths *per step* and basically pulling one of the guys up to the top. It was miserable, and I had a decision to make. I had to commit here. Either make it to the top or die trying. Okay . . . onward.

It wasn't until another half-hour of suffering when something dawned on me. Why was I being so stupid? I remembered the story of the Taoist master who linked the energy of his dantien to his disciples and pulled them across a raging river. This was the story that got me into this mess! If this Taoist magic stuff really worked, then I should be able to use it now!

After a little bit of thought, I figured that if a master could link his dantien to others' and create a connection, then he was doing so by anchoring the connection with his mind, or *shen*. I figured I'd do it a little differently. I basically assigned my lower dantien to the very top of that mountain and created a strong connection with it. I then breathed down to my lower dantien and focused my energy there. Once the connection was in place, I simply "created" gravity between the two points. I allowed myself to "fall up the hill" as my lower dantien was being tugged by a strong connection with the top of the mountain.

Next thing I knew, my rope was getting tight, and I found that I was pulling away from the Swiss guys behind me. The guide (who must have been part mountain goat) was quite surprised by my sudden burst of energy. Realizing that I was linked by ropes to the other two behind me, I attempted to do what the master in the story did. Whether I actually did it or they were being encouraged by my tugging of the rope, I don't know. All I know is that I was suddenly leading the charge up the mountain. Once at the top, I felt an incredible sense of heat in my lower dantien as I literally walked straight into an ice-covered rock with my dantien leading. I had to release the gravity consciously before it would let go.

We sat for a while and reveled at our accomplishment. More important, we reveled at how the world looked from that high. It seemed that we could *see* the curvature of the atmosphere above us. We stayed for a short while and then quickly got down to base camp, each step getting lighter and easier all the way down. Getting up there was nice, but the real lesson for me was finding the power and magnitude of my lower dantien.

The Different Types of Qi Gong Practice

There is a yin and a yang aspect to everything, including the actual energetic practice. We studied the various types of energy earlier. Now, some of that information will come to light a bit more. The nutritive qi and the defensive qi are the main types of energy running through our body. They tend to our cells and service our myriad physiological needs. For these types of qi, there are practices designed to emphasize one or the other. In fact, there are also practices designed to enhance shen, or spirit, as well as other internal practices designed to cultivate and refine essence and awaken the spirit within. Here are the designations of the various qi gong practices:

- *Wei gong:* This practice concentrates on the exterior energy (wei qi), which is responsible for health, immunity, and the defense of the system against pathogens and disease. It is designed to route energy to these external "force fields" and to create an energetic barrier that protects the internal organs from outside invasion.

- *Qi gong:* This is a general term for the practices that bolster the nutritive qi and that also support the defensive qi.

It increases flow to the different systems and provides the body with the necessary boost it needs to nourish and heal itself. Qi gong is the most balanced approach; however, it needs to be modified depending on the circumstances of the individual or for progressing into deeper work.

- *Nei gong:* This is considered the higher alchemical practice that is taught in the temples; it involves a great deal of dedication. Nei gong emphasizes the cultivation and preservation of essence (sexual abstinence mixed with specific practices) so that it can be further condensed and refined to qi and shen. Nei gong leads to the formation of the Light Body and is what has been passed down by the famous Taoist "immortals." It takes many months of qi gong practice with mental and emotional reconciliation before nei gong is considered safe.

- *Shen gong:* This practice applies to the cultivation of the attention and, specifically, the cultivation of the psychic senses that help us perceive energetic rhythms universally. It aids in clairvoyance, clairaudience, long-distance healing, astral travel, and psionics/mind control. This is obviously high-level stuff, but this practice should not be considered the most important. As far as I'm concerned, this stuff is "cute," but the real gold is in the nei gong, which effectuates personal transformation. Shen gong is often taught to priests who need to intervene in crises, heal ailments, and perform exorcisms. It is an important part of the knowledge of the Tao, but the danger in the West is in how people glorify the "powers," which can then serve as a dangerous ego trap.

Just like the emphasis we put on getting the physical body healthy and fit, it is important to start here with the foundations of qi gong and work our way up. This means working diligently on our stance, which will help ground our energy and give us "roots." Stances develop the lower dantien and strengthen the wei (or defensive) qi. Once we build a strong foundation, we can really begin to reap the powerful benefits of this practice. From here, we learn about the mysteries of the Tao and become more self-aware.

Words of Caution

We need wax for a candle to be a candle and to serve its purpose. Thus, the practice begins with foundational work that will strengthen our muscles, bones, energy flow, and resolve. We are blessed to have these systems available to us, and it is truly fortunate that the air of secrecy that originally surrounded these arts has changed in our age. That being said, though, there is work to do, and shortcuts are dangerous.

Taoism is about maintaining balance and harmonizing the polarity consciousness that has infected the minds of our culture. Just like you can't "power nap" each night for an hour instead of getting a full night's sleep, you can't not do the work. Sure, you can get away with those power naps for a few days or weeks (likely with the help of stimulants and drugs), but you'll quickly burn out. Again, look at this behavior bathed in the full light of what we have learned about aversions and cravings. Look at how some people will do anything to avoid feeling their past and the nonsense they will resort to in order to run from themselves. This is not healthy behavior, and we are here to correct it. The way is the training.

I have been practicing and teaching in Southern California for decades now, and I have encountered a great many "hungry ghosts." These spiritual shoppers are looking for a quick fix and will do something that is convenient, but they are not willing to put in any real work. This is especially true if the work challenges them to face the content in their shadows. Similar to the discussion in the previous chapter on eating habits, I find it very telling to see how a student engages in a practice and with what level of commitment. When someone is given a specific diet that avoids foods that they are *allergic to* (validated by testing) and they fail to comply because it is "too hard," then that is a telling characteristic of a zombie—someone who is completely powerless to face him- or herself. I see much of the same with people who want the "fuzzy" stuff with the qi gong but are unwilling to do the foundation-building work. They are impatient and will get nowhere. I'm here to help, but I can't do the work for you. I *will* point you in the right direction, though.

So, take a deep breath, and let's get into the training!

7

QI GONG EXERCISES

If a man knows the method to nourish the breath,
he is able to become an immortal.

TAO TSANG, Taoist Canon (translated by Jane Huang)

ooking at pictures of exercises in a book is not the ideal way to learn in this modern age of web streaming. Actually, no media format is ideal for learning qi gong, as these traditions have been passed down through *direct transmission* over thousands of years. In fact, my grand master prohibits the use of video cameras with the Taoist nei gong system of our lineage, where oral and personal transmissions are the only means allowed. Other traditions are a bit more lax. Moving sequenced sets are obviously harder to illustrate in a book than standing or seated static exercises, but the real key is to convey the work accurately so that the reader can learn it and practice *correctly*.

In light of this, after a good deal of thought and meditation, I have developed a program that I feel addresses the fundamentals of practice and really sets things up correctly for your energy practice. You will learn three traditional exercises in this chapter that will get you well on your way to better health, stamina, and energy flow.

I want nothing less than *complete transformation* for you. Holding that thinking in mind, it is important for you to practice all the exercises in this book. This means the physical practice (diet, exercise, sleep, and basic lifestyle modification); the qi gong practice in this chapter (all three exercises); and the mental, emotional, and spiritual practices that follow. I have boiled energy cultivation down into a cohesive and effective system; all it takes is for you to plug into it. You do the work, and you reap the rewards. The formula is that easy.

EXERCISE 1
The Silk Weaver's Exercise (Wei Gong/Qi Gong)

This particular sequence is a health set that helps open up and dilate the meridians. It is of Buddhist origins and has been taught for years as the quintessential health set of the qi gong tradition. It is to be done three times—two moving repetitions and one with the eyes closed doing the entire thing through visualization.

This set is a moving set; in order to preserve the integrity of the motions, I'd like for you to go to the following link to see it: SoundsTrue.com/inner-alchemy/bonus. This site provides unlimited free access for you to view the exercise to make sure you are doing it correctly. All the fundamentals are important for this exercise, including having the tip of the tongue touch the roof of the mouth and having a feeling of heaviness in the lower body. Please spend some time learning this and burning it into your body's memory so you can practice it anywhere you may be.

Learning sequenced movements is an important practice that not only makes you more aware but also helps develop the brain and nervous system.

EXERCISE 2
The Shaolin Standing Form (Qi Gong/Strength Building)

This set comes from the Shaolin tradition and is incredibly challenging at first for many people, as most people in the modern age have weak postural muscles and are not accustomed to deep lower abdominal breathing. These deep stances help build resolve and help develop a powerful connection with the lower dantien. The hand postures help open energy flow through the shoulders (where many of us have trapped energy) and through axillary arteries.

Try to stay in these stances for a designated amount of time and try to maintain your stances consistently. This may be difficult at first, but you will quickly find that you can do more and more with sustained practice. It is okay to feel challenged in your leg muscles, but do not force your way through joint pain. You can turn your feet slightly outward if your knees bother you. Keep the tongue touching the roof of the mouth, and breathe in and out of the lower abdomen for all the exercises taught henceforth.

If you begin to feel light-headed during the early stages of this practice, it is likely due to the massive energy reserves being released. Just have a seat and begin again when you've gained your composure. It is perfectly natural to feel a rush of energy rise to the head during this exercise.

Since this is a static exercise, examine each posture individually in this section. Pick a designated amount of time to stay in each posture and increase the time as your proficiency develops. Thirty seconds to a minute per posture is enough for most people when they start. Try to add thirty seconds per posture per week if you can, as this will quickly propel you into a very strong practice. The energy that gets freed up in your system will feel great and will serve as an encouragement to keep practicing.

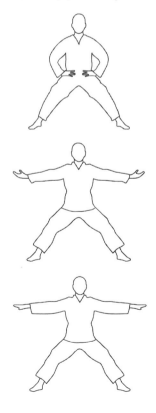

OPENING STANCE   SQUARE HORSE
Stand with even weight distribution between both legs. Keep your head up straight with your hands at waist level.

STANCE 1   PALMS UP, RESISTING UPWARD
Imagine a very heavy weight on top of each palm. Resist to keep them up.

STANCE 2   PALMS DOWN, RESISTING DOWNWARD
Imagine a force pushing up from the earth against your palms. Work to stay in position.

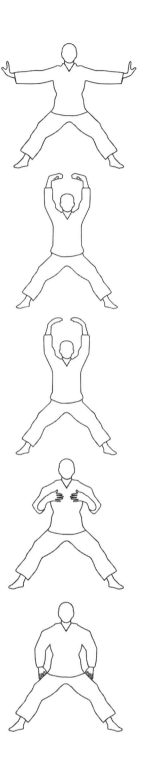

STANCE 3   FINGERTIPS UP, PRESSING OUTWARD

Now the imaginary force is coming in from the sides, like elevator doors closing. Hold outward.

STANCE 4   PALMS UP, PRESSING AGAINST THE SKY

Now the imaginary force is bearing down on you. Use dynamic tension to resist against it.

STANCE 5   PALMS DOWN, POURING ENERGY INTO THE HEAD

Let your palms rain energy back down onto your head and body.

STANCE 6   PALMS FACING CHEST, GATHERING ENERGY IN THE HEART

Feel the energy swirl between your palms and your torso. Gather energy into your heart.

STANCE 7   PALMS FLAT BEHIND BACK WITH FINGERS POINTING FORWARD AND PALMS FACING DOWN, CONNECTING WITH THE GROUND

Round out the elbows as you feel your kidneys fill up with energy. Resist a force pushing up from the earth with palms flat.

STANCE 8 PALMS TOGETHER, GATHERING ENERGY IN THE HEART

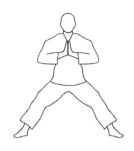

Rest in prayer position and allow the energy to gather in your heart.

As I mentioned, this series of exercise is from the Shaolin kung fu tradition. It is "hard work," which is a wonderful thing, as it creates a good habit of allowing you to push through certain blockages and trains you to deal with muscle pain (and burning!) with equanimity. Remember, Shaolin is the birthplace of the Zen tradition. When you put this art into actual practice, it is the physical body's reflection of the mental practice of nonreacting to aversions and cravings. The Shaolin system trains the "bodymind" as a unified complex; proficiency in this training leads to excellent meditation skills.

EXERCISE 3
The Triple Burner Exercise (Wei Gong/Qi Gong)

This exercise uses a series of dynamic standing postures with breathwork, just like the previous exercise, but it also incorporates another layer of sophistication, which is the practice of guided visualization. The triple burner exercise is an effective health set that teaches you to use your shen to guide your energy to certain places within the body. With sustained focus, you will learn to heal yourself and to bring the light of awareness to different body parts. This is your first venture in guiding qi internally; the mastery of this principle will allow you to move into higher principles of nei gong.

BASIC STANCE

Stand in a basic wu chi posture: The feet are shoulder-width apart. The hands are off to the sides with a bit of space under each armpit, palms facing behind you. This practice uses what is called "four point" balancing, where you balance your weight on the balls and heels of each foot. Touch the tip of the tongue to the roof of the mouth and breathe in nose and out nose to the lower dantien.

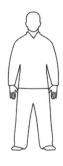

POSTURE 1   UPPER BURNER

Organs to clear: heart, lungs, pericardium, glands in the throat

- Hold your hands in the "tree" position up in front of your chest.

- Keep breathing in nose and out nose to the lower dantien.

- Stay with your four-point stance throughout this entire exercise.

- Start breathing to your palms and feel a white light emanating from the center of your palms into your upper chest.

- Simultaneously, reflect this light back from the upper chest to push against your palms.

- Feel the exchange of energy between the palms and the chest. Shift your attention to this area but keep breathing to the lower dantien.

- Stay here in this posture until you feel that all the energy in this region is fully cleared before moving to the next posture. When you can sense only clean energy and white light, that is when you're done.

POSTURE 2   MIDDLE BURNER

Organs to clear: stomach, spleen, liver, gallbladder, upper intestine, pancreas

- Move your hands slightly lower to the level of the lower sternum.

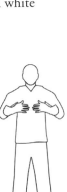

- Continue the same practice as in the first posture, until you feel that this level is completely clear of any blockages.

- Remember to inundate the area with pure white light and to really focus on the exchange between the palms and the torso.

POSTURE 3   LOWER BURNER

Organs to clear: kidneys (in the back), bladder, intestines, sexual organs

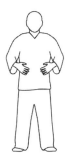

- Move your hands slightly lower to the level of the navel.

- Continue the same practice until you feel that this level is completely clear of any blockages.

- Really focus and clear as many energetic blockages as you can find in the gut region.

POSTURE 4   KIDNEYS

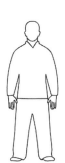

- Move your hands behind the back with palms flat and facing the ground behind the kidneys.

- Connect the light coming from your palms with the earth.

- On the inhale (in nose), visualize liquid white light coming up from your feet and your palms all the way to the crown of your head.

- On the exhale (out nose), push this energy back down into the earth through the palms and feet.

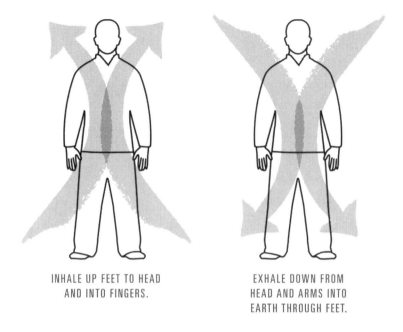

INHALE UP FEET TO HEAD
AND INTO FINGERS.

EXHALE DOWN FROM
HEAD AND ARMS INTO
EARTH THROUGH FEET.

- Continue to draw energy up to the crown on the inhale and back down into the earth on the exhale for several breaths.

- When you feel like your body is free and clear of any blocked energies, take a long exhale out of the mouth and move to the closing sequence.

CLOSING SEQUENCE   SELF-MASSAGE

- Rub from the backs of your shoulders (one at a time) down the outside of the arm to the pinky with the opposite hand and then back up the thumb side into the chest.

- Circle and rub your heart region and then your lower dantien.

- Rub your kidney region on your back with both palms.

- Rub down the backs of both legs while bending forward and then rub up the front while standing upright again.

- Tap your lower dantien (three finger-widths below your navel) three times with both hands.

With continued practice of this set, you will develop clarity of mind and a clean energy field. This is a critical skill to help you grow and understand your essential nature. When you stop identifying with the "noise" and clean your energy field, you become more and more aware of who you truly are. This is one of the most liberating things you can do for yourself.

Sequencing

In an ideal situation, it would be best to practice exercises 1 and 2 in the morning (outdoors in fresh air if possible) at least thirty to sixty minutes after a short walk to get the blood moving but before breakfast. Yes, this means getting up earlier, but the benefits are simply priceless. Exercise 3 can be done at any point throughout the day but preferably before 9:00 p.m. Do not perform exercise 3 too close to bedtime as it may stimulate you too much and cause insomnia. It is actually a great exercise to do around 3:00 or 4:00 p.m., when your energy may start to fade. Just a few minutes in a short set is better than nothing, and you'll feel great. Play with it and see what works best for you.

Qi Gong Rule: Do not eat sixty minutes before training and at least thirty minutes after training. This may be difficult in the mornings especially, but it is important to observe. Here's what I have done for years: I wake up, go for a run or brisk walk, do my practice for thirty minutes or so, then jump in the shower and go through my preparatory morning routine. By then, I'm ready to eat anyhow, and things have settled. When you are ready, eat a healthy breakfast and be on your way.

If you make it a point to get all three exercises in every day, you will start to feel a profound difference very quickly. It is important to note that a great deal of stagnant and trapped energy will be released throughout this process. Some people feel dizzy and/or light-headed in the first couple of weeks (especially in exercise 2). Take it slowly and work your way up to greater difficulty. More time and deeper stances are where you should aim to be, but all within reason. Remember, Taoism is about balance. There's good stress and unhealthy stress on the system. You want to walk that razor's edge and stay right in the middle—pushing yourself to evolve and grow without overstepping your limits. When you commit to making it your daily practice, the pressure is off, and you can keep moving the marker forward every day.

A good example of this steady progress is kung fu high-jumping training. When a young monk starts his training, he is given a baby stalk of corn to plant and care for. His assignment is to jump over this stalk ten times daily with both feet. He does this religiously for months on end until he realizes that he is clearing a few feet with a vertical jump! This is how your practice will progress. Follow the instructions carefully and integrate the exercises from this chapter in order to make the training complete. Remember, you don't want to "pick and choose" what's most convenient for you, because that usually implies that you are acting out of trance and avoiding something that makes you uncomfortable.

8

MENTAL PRACTICE

The basic difference between an ordinary man and a Warrior is that
the Warrior sees everything as a challenge whereas the ordinary
man sees everything as either a blessing or a curse.

CARLOS CASTANEDA, *The Teachings of Don Juan*

etting the physical body healthy through lifestyle and activating the
proper flow of energy through qi gong are essential steps to waking
up and snapping out of our trancelike slumber. However, we have to
maintain the correct mindset in our training or we'll be running around in
circles for a long time. It is futile to bring up the amount of energy running
through our system while continuing to play the same games of our past.
If we don't wake up and clearly recognize our habits and tendencies of old,
then we may as well not even start. Simply put, there are a number of places
and circumstances where we tend to "leak" our energy, and these holes need
to be plugged up. Recall from part I when I spoke of polarity and the
tendency of the human mind to channel energy into the opposite polarity of what we are feeling. Essentially, we are channeling our energy into
situations that we are uncomfortable with and reinforcing them through
our ignorance of how our energy systems work. The point is that we really
don't have anything to "do" here, per se, other than accepting reality as it
is in every moment. Our judgment (or our aversions and cravings) of any
given item or situation is where we literally breathe life into our lack of
acceptance of these things, and this is what births our monsters.

In this book, we have come to understand the nature of how we create such harmful mental karma; thus, we are now poised to practice just the opposite. We are going to learn something that is at first very difficult to do for the human mind, but it is an important step in our journey. This is to do *nothing at all*. As mentioned in part I, the concept of karma is simply the action that we take. This applies to the mental, emotional, spiritual, and physical. Anytime we "move" to do or create something, we are generating karma. Every time we react to a given thought or statement, our mental waves reflect this reaction to the edge of the universe and back. Instead of being listening stations for the symphony of the cosmic Tao, we are broadcasting stations for the reflections of our shadows, spewing chaos and noise into the universe.

The ancient Taoists spoke of the concept of the *yi*, or the intellect, creating a disturbance in the heart. The disruptions of the mind manifest as an invading space that slowly grows and eventually nudges out the shen of the heart. When the shen doesn't have a house to settle in, it cannot reside in the body, and we perish. Therefore, a big part of the Taoist immortality practice is the clearing of this disrupted yi from the heart.

Taoist Mental Practice

This exercise will start to create an understanding of the overactive role your mind plays in every instant of your life. Practice it daily in silence and then take it into your day-to-day life. The goal is to be constantly practicing this at all times, day and night. You may think to yourself, *How am I going to get anything done then?* The answer is simple: you'll get more done efficiently when you are not blowing away all your energy into chaos. *Trust. Practice.*

PREPARATORY STEPS

- Sit in a quiet place with your spine straight and body relaxed. A cushion on the floor is ideal, but a firm chair will also work—just don't lean back in it.

- Rest your hands on your knees with the thumb and index fingers touching, palms up.

- Take ten breaths into your lower dantien (three finger-widths below your navel), in nose and out nose.

- Settle into your breath and relax your mind.

BEGIN THE PRACTICE

- Your only action item in this practice is to ask yourself, *What am I doing right now?*

- Whatever it is that you are mentally engaged in, simply *stop doing that* and relax.

- Stay in this state of *inaction* but constantly pose the same question to yourself: *What am I doing right now?*

- You'll find that you tend to get pretty busy doing *something* all of the time. Don't get upset with yourself and think of yourself as a failure—welcome to the nature of the mind! We all have this noise, and we are all constantly jumping into the mental ring with it and fighting it to exhaustion.

- Again: *What am I doing right now?* Do this for ten to fifteen minutes at a time at first and extend sitting time as you progress.

If we are going to practice and cultivate *inaction*, which is the opposite of *doing*, then what do we do? There is only one *action* allowed in this exercise, and that is the last action that bridges us into the realm of inaction.

Taking the Practice with You

With continued practice, you will learn to become more and more aware of this tendency to always be doing something, and you will understand how much *effort* you are putting into this nonsense all the time! The only reason any of us feel any "lack" of energy is that we are spending 99 percent of our time *leaking* our energy on this freight train of nonsense that's constantly running through our head.

Once you get a sense of how this practice works, simply program your subconscious mind to continue to ask it of yourself throughout your day.

True meditation is a state of being; it is not what you do for twenty minutes on your cushion! Let this practice function as a self-diagnostic or correctional program that keeps pulling your awareness back to what it is you are actually doing in the present moment. You will find that, with time, it is tremendously liberating, and you will learn to relax more and more into your *intact* energy field.

Western students often ask me about the principle of inaction. The general theme of their questions is, "If I were to relax and do nothing all day, then how could I perform my job and feed my family? How do I reconcile this paradox?" To them I often share the following story:

There is a famous tale of a Zen monastery in the mountains where an enormous boulder rolled down into the grounds after a storm. A number of monks were outside fretting over it when the master came out to inquire about all of the noise and fuss they were making. Without giving it another thought, the master simply picked up the huge boulder and carried it off to the side of the plaza. Unable to believe their eyes, the monks asked their master how he was able to perform such an extraordinary feat, and his reply was simple: "I simply relaxed as deeply as I exerted and lifted."

Don't worry about what you insist on getting done! If it needs to be done, it'll happen naturally at the right time. We spend 99 percent of our time and energy playing out scenarios or anticipating an action instead of relaxing and doing it naturally. We're so tired by then that most of us can't even perform the action right when it is time. Practice these exercises and don't fall for your mental trance arguments. You'll be better than fine.

9

EMOTIONAL PRACTICE

If a person's mind is not excited with thoughts,
there is no coming and no going, there is no exiting and no entering,
then (the Spirit) constantly abides naturally (inside).

TAO TSANG, Taoist Canon, Vol. IV (translated by Jane Huang)

Having set up a precedent for our understanding of reality and the nature of our suffering, we can now bridge into the healing of the soul. The "horizontal axis" of the soul is where we have stored many lessons and a great deal of energy that remains trapped and stagnant. It is this trapped energy that feeds our internal "demons" and the behaviors that plague us so much. But it doesn't have to be this way.

With the framework of self-care, qi gong, and mental awareness practice that we have just learned, we are now poised to delve into the "darkness" of the shadow and start the alchemical process in full force. Finding the "lead," which we will turn into "gold," is easy—we simply need to discover the things that bother us the most in any given day and start with them. It may be a reaction to our spouse's dilly-dallying or maybe the behavior of a certain co-worker. Whatever it is that upsets us, chances are it isn't anything new to us.

As mentioned in part I, we start to create the spin in the bolstered energy fields of our attachments, and, in doing so, our fields take on other similar issues. They fall into families of issues by topic and class. We start with what Alfred Korzybski called the original event, and then we keep branching out and expanding from there, moving further and further into levels of "abstraction."[1] We get further away from the essential truth of the original event, and we start to create story lines for ourselves to make it okay. The more this goes on, the more energy we pump into this artificial field. The more energy we put in, the more it seems utterly impossible for us to penetrate this mutated, powerful field and face the truth. We create monsters out of undesirable events, and we feed them until they own us.

So, here's the way out. First and foremost, we have to stop the bleeding. This requires *awareness* of these patterns and *forgiveness* in the moment. Using the mental practice taught in the previous chapter, we should be constantly scanning to see what mess we're about to get involved in and stop it right there. Once we get the hang of it, we invariably find that we're about to go down a very familiar road with a given subject. This is where the attention of the shen (which is housed in the heart) comes in. We have detected a given behavior or karmic action from an old theme, and we have *recognized* that we are about to go into some old trance behavior. What can we do?

We must first acknowledge this behavior, and then, focusing on our heart, we must immediately go into *forgiving* whomever, whatever, and however anyone was involved. Far from the polarity consciousness of our reactive mind, the heart holds our personal connection with the primordial Tao. It is our true state of being, prior to the separation of yin and yang. Once we tap into this with the energy of forgiveness, we can hold it in our heart and consciously *reclaim* our power from this event or memory. We do this by understanding the fundamental split that took place in our mind and then pulling back the energy we deposited into the opposite pole.

For instance, say your father was abusive to you as a child, and you are still harboring ill will toward him, even though he's now a broken-down old man. The typical behavior you automatically default to when he calls is to get very short and cool with him. You could be out at the pool with the family having the perfect day, and then *he* calls. Your breath shortens, your pulse speeds up, and you are suddenly in a very different space. What's the first thing to do? *Recognize* what it is that you're doing right then. *You* are the one getting revved up, *you* are the one raising your blood pressure, and *you* are the one lowering your voice and going from smile to frown over this. So, what then? *Stop it.* Recognize the unconscious behavior and then stop it in that instant.

Now, yes, I understand that's easier said than done, but that's because there is such a massive *charge* around your relationship with your father. The energy is stored up like a balloon about to burst. But this is where you must *change* your typical behavior or else you'll feed even more negative energy into your chapter of "father." This is where you drop into your heart; forgive him for whatever he has done right there and then; and, with the energy neutralized (in the moment), begin to see the pattern for what it is. Every time he comes up in your thought field, a whole slew of emotions race in and get you all fired up. But now, instead of channeling daggers into the aversion of your father, channel forgiveness to the man himself. Forgive him, forgive his behavior, forgive yourself, and forgive the situation. Thank him for the lessons he has given you and for the opportunity to be more loving. *Understand* that his behavior (whatever it was he did or still does) is a product of an imbalance. He was (is) acting out on his demons, and they, in turn, have *infected* you. Do not accept them! The only way you can get infected is if you buy into and then co-create that imbalanced energy yourself. A powerful thing to say in this instance is, "This is not my energy, these are not my demons, and I do not accept this into my field."

Having withdrawn our energy from our typical patterns, we may now focus on the original split that created the charge around this field and apply our knowledge to actively target and mend that schism. Remember, all movement and life began with the split into yin and yang. Therefore, our polarization of the energy related to any given event is what gave it an initial charge and brought it to life. Our recognition of this allows us to withdraw our attention from this polarity and reunite the energy as a whole. We focus on the item in our mind's eye and simply feel where we've been misdirecting all our energy. And remember, it's *our* power, so it should be easy to find. Once we reclaim it, we can pull it back into our lower dantien and then seal it in there mentally. From that point, we can *watch* the energy field of the original issue collapse, and then we can *continue* to forgive it until it is completely gone.

In the example of dealing with your dad, go back to the first time you recall him treating you that way and forgive that moment. Use the mental practice to trace around the timeline and clean and clear with forgiveness. You should be able to heal any particular issue within one to three times of following this practice. The more you pay attention and the more focused you remain, the quicker it'll be done. If you catch yourself leaking more energy into the shadow when you think about a subject, simply trace your way back to the root of it again. Like the pull of gravity, follow the cord of energy flow back to the original event and confront it there. This is the quickest way to heal these attachments. They don't want to live in the shadow; all discordant energy wants to return to the Source. Think of it like a homecoming—pull all your fragmented pieces back into yourself.

CLINICAL ENCOUNTERS   Letting Go

Emily came to me for acupuncture after years of trying pretty much everything. She had seen medical doctors, chiropractors, psychotherapists, hypnotherapists, and faith healers. Nothing had worked for her panic attacks. I immediately got the sense that she was a "shopper"—the type of patient who wants you to tell them what they want to hear. They'll accept help only on *their* terms. She had smut on everyone she'd seen before me, but *I* was going to be her savior; *I* was the hero who was going to help her this time.

I stood up to walk out of the room. I had been here too many times, and I was not about to be another in a long string of "failures" for her. I kindly told her that I wasn't going to be able to meet her expectations and that she shouldn't waste her time and money with me. This infuriated her! She begged and cried and pleaded that I help her, so I told her that the only way I could do *anything* was if she let me in. My terms were simple: we were going to find the original trauma and heal it by feeling it. Somehow I got through to her, and two hours later, she walked out and never had another panic attack again.

The power of honesty and the power of actually "going there" cannot be underestimated. We traced her discordant energy back to its original event, and it was a cleanup job from there. I taught her how to watch for emotional triggers in the future, and she was elated to have found such helpful knowledge that she could apply herself. It was also a powerful moment for me because it reinforced two things: (1) This stuff really works and is very powerful, and (2) nobody can do it for you; you must do it yourself. I helped Emily see the problem and taught her how to release it. She healed the wound, and that made her whole. It really helped me understand my role as a physician: to teach is to heal.

Taoist Five Elemental Magic

Once you fully understand this practice, you can instantly heal emotional issues and absorb your power back from your shadow. The more practice you get, the better you will become at this, and the easier and more enjoyable it will be. The next step is not always necessary, but it certainly is helpful—it is a tried-and-true practice of Taoist alchemists designed for the internal healing of organs and emotions using the five elements. Refer to table 9.1, which shows these elemental correspondences, to reinforce your understanding of this science.

Taking this matrix and assessing which emotions are challenging you in a given situation, you can then visualize the color and chant the sound of that organ and focus on them. Notice that the yin and yang organs have different sounds associated with them. Search your energy field and determine which one you feel needs the attention, and then focus on it. Of course, you can do this separately, focusing on either sound or color, or you can do both simultaneously, using both color and sound.

Let's go through an example. Let's say you are dealing with a lot of anger right now. In this case, visualize focusing *green light* (imagine the color of fresh grass growing in the spring) over your liver along the right side of the rib cage. Inhale the green light to the area and chant the organ sound *Shh . . . u* (the first sound drops into the second) on the exhale.

TABLE 9.1   FIVE ELEMENT SOUNDS

ELEMENT	FIRE	EARTH	METAL	WATER	WOOD
Yin Organ(s)	Heart, pericardium	Spleen	Lungs	Kidneys	Liver
Yang Organ(s)	Small intestine, triple burner	Stomach	Large intestine	Bladder	Gall Bladder
Emotions	Mania, lack of joy in life	Worry	Grief	Fear	Anger
Healing Color	Rich red	Vibrant green	Sunshine yellow	Pure white	Dark blue
Yin Healing Sound	Haa	Huu	Shh	Fuu . . . u	Shh . . . u
Yang Healing Sound	Kee-D	Hoo-R	Hoo-D	Yaa-R	Jaa-R

Do this softly and repeat it over and over until you feel that the energy is cleansed. Imagine the light as a "puffy cloud" around the organ on the inhale and *condense* it into the organ on the exhale while making the healing sound. If you'd like, you could also use the same green light over the gallbladder, but this time you would chant *Jaa-R* on the exhale.

You can cycle through all the elements to conduct a "maintenance" round or simply focus in on an afflicted element. This exercise is particularly effective for problems with the internal organs. Simply go through the exercise and allow the pure color and/or sound of the element to cleanse and heal the organ. This example of "resonant tuning" allows you to hold pathological or imbalanced vibrations against their correct archetypal "gold standards" and give them the space to self-correct.

Once you feel proficient at this, you can apply the same practice with the generating and controlling cycles mentioned earlier (see figures 4.10 and 4.11). In the generating cycle, you can follow the arrows and heal the elements upstream or downstream from your afflicted element to help bring balance to your system. Let's take the previous example of anger—a disharmonious wood element. You have focused on the healing with color and sound, but you still feel edgy and frustrated. So you feed the "mother" element of water and focus dark blue light to the kidneys while chanting *Fuu . . . u* on the exhale. This may bring the necessary healing to the wood element, which has been drained over several years of emotional turmoil. Remember, since everything is in a cycle, things upstream or downstream may be affecting what you are feeling right now. Use your intuition to scan internally and *see* where the attention needs to be focused.

Using the controlling cycle (figure 4.11), you could also support the metal element to check or control the wood element if you need further assistance. Do this by focusing white light on the lungs while chanting *Shh* on the exhale.

Now, there's also a more advanced variant that you may want to try. When scanning your consciousness and uprooting old emotional trance content, *feel* this energy and determine whether it is in excess or in deficiency. Is there too much energy overflowing in this system, or is there not enough, making the system crave more? Once you've made your determination, you can nourish the "mother" using the generating cycle for a deficient case (in the anger/wood example, the mother is water), *or* you can nourish the controlling element (called the grandfather in Taoist medicine) in a case of excess (again, in the anger/wood example, the grandfather is metal). This practice is a bit more advanced and requires a certain degree of self-awareness and deeper focus. If you do not feel comfortable with your determination of which way to balance, you can stay with the first exercise of bringing light to the afflicted element. Once you get the hang of that, you can work your way into the more advanced techniques. I encourage you not to worry about whether you are doing it "right" or "wrong." Bringing pure, undifferentiated light and a healing sound can only heal an imbalance; worst-case scenario, you will have healed the wrong organ or element system. There is no downside for this, and the organ will thank you for it!

How to Do the Emotional Practice

What is absolutely important before starting this form of mental and emotional cleaning is to thoroughly orient yourself in time and space. This is done very easily out of the middle dantien, or heart center (which is in the middle of chest, as opposed to the actual heart organ, which is shifted slightly to the left). Here is the process:

- Sit or stand facing the south.

- Close your eyes and center your awareness in your heart center.

- Focus a beam of light from your heart center up through your crown and to the center of the universe.

- Send another beam down through your perineum to the center of the Earth. (All beams start at the heart center.)

- Now, you will send beams out in all four cardinal directions.

- Start in front of you to the south and out to infinity.

- Next, send another beam through your back to the north.

- Next, send one out your left side to the east.

- And finally, send a beam out the right side of your heart center to the west.

Once you have linked up to the six directions through your heart, you are poised to perform your inner alchemical work and have it register more effectively. You can do this quickly from wherever you are as a quick centering exercise. If you don't have a compass and are not oriented, simply say "south" in your mind's eye, and your shen will know what to do. Make sure you send out beams in all six directions, as this is what literally "parks" your shen at a "zip code" or exact coordinate point in the universe. This anchoring in the six directions is a critical component to all alchemical systems and is one that we will come back to (using the upper dantien) in our more advanced studies.

So, here is how to do the emotional practice to clean out any impedance or patterns:

- Orient yourself in time and space by connecting to the six directions.

- Recognize the pattern through your mental awareness training and stop yourself before you do it again.

- Forgive the perpetrator, situation, or conduct.

- Withdraw your energy from your typical response pattern.

- Bring balance to the yin-yang split by withdrawing your energy from any further creation of the field.

- Continue to forgive and balance the pattern in your mind's eye, and watch the field around it "deflate" and lose its power.

- Reabsorb this power into your lower dantien.

- Link up with the six directions through the middle dantien again.

- Practice the Taoist five elemental magic as needed.

- Go back to scanning with your awareness for any similar "threads" of discordant energy and apply the same practice to them.

Please remember that this is a *process* and that there is plenty of junk to work through. Once you get into the game and start to understand it, you'll get better and better at it. It becomes fun (believe it or not), and you will feel incredibly liberated the further you go with it. Keep releasing trapped energy and remember to absorb it back into your field. With time, you'll have more power and focus at your disposal to engage further into this process.

Once you are feeling better, you will naturally notice imbalances and shadow energy trapped in other people. When you see this, come back to your own center and heal the energy *in yourself.* Your connection with the Tao (linking up with the six directions) will facilitate this process. Allow your heart to feel compassion for the plight of others and then heal whatever you see in yourself. There's never a dull moment for an alchemist, and you'll find that boredom will be a thing of the past. Hurry up—the world needs you!

10

SPIRITUAL PRACTICE

The Kingdom of Spirit is embodied in my flesh.

HERMES TRISMEGISTUS, The Pattern on the Trestleboard

The essence of Taoist spiritual practice is one of *purification* and *reduction*. I mentioned earlier that qi gong is a "subtraction" process in that it helps take away blockages *against* the free flow of energy moving through us. This is an important understanding that underscores our connection with nature. This relationship with nature is not so much an abstract feeling that we tap into when we look out over the Grand Canyon as much as it is who we are. We are One with all that is around us, and the perception of separation can be likened to the proverbial "fall" from the Garden of Eden. This intimate and personal interweaving of ourselves and our environment is the foundation of the Taoist understanding of reality and is the source of our ultimate liberation.

Once we shake out all our faulty belief systems and trance-inspired ideas about ourselves, we can begin to encounter the wonderment of who we truly are, and it is nothing less than amazing. The problem is, in line with polarity consciousness, we tend to move *away* from our center to find ourselves. We ask around and look up to an abstract concept of "heaven," seeking peace and salvation. But that is the exact opposite direction, and it marks the primordial disconnection from the Tao. Healing this tendency is the most powerful act in which we can participate. It brings peace and understanding. It brings us back to our inner nature.

In this chapter, we will further study the framework of the five elements as the model with which we will work. We will also learn a certain purification process under each element. I encourage you to practice these as often as possible. At first, things may seem awkward as we look through the goggles of our trance mentality. Keeping our focus on the practice, however, will allow us to discover that we are more and more interested in these practices of inner discovery and less inclined to seek out distractions and sedatives in our outer lives.

The Spiritual Purification Practices of the Five Elements

In chapter 4, we discussed the relationship of the five elements. Now we're going study each element individually. You may want to review the five element correspondences in table 4.2.

EARTH

The purification practice for the earth element is intimately related to the food that we eat. In previous chapters, we discussed the types, quantity, and timing of the food that we choose; now we're going to examine the *quality* and *source* of these foods.

Everything that is material has an energetic and spiritual nature (as discussed in part I). Everything—animal, plants, and even minerals—also carries consciousness. In fact, if it exists, it shares in the universal consciousness of which we are a part. So, the source of our nutrition really dictates the quality of energy we ingest. This was rarely a problem in the ancient world, as food sources were pure and directly extracted from a healthy environment. It has changed in modernity, however, with agribusiness and urbanization. We now face a good deal of toxicity, hormones, and unhappy energy in what we eat. Livestock that are raised pumped up with steroids and hormones and that are then brutally butchered carry a distinct energy pattern that is of a very low vibration. Grains are mass produced with pesticides and processed by mindless people in plants and then boxed and refortified. Most grains have been genetically modified in order to produce better yields and are devoid of life force, and many of us are having trouble assimilating them. If we are going to follow the axiom "we are what we eat," then we'd better be eating pure, natural, high-quality, cruelty-free foods. Doing so has a direct effect on our energy and spirit. It is best to get locally grown fruits and vegetables that are organically grown and are treated with *love*. This critical aspect is often overlooked in our culture. Meat is a racy topic and has generated much debate for decades. If you do eat meat, *never* buy traditional meats; make sure the meat is from animals raised in a healthy fashion—that is, free range and cruelty-free.

Reverence thus becomes the centerpiece of the earth element spiritual purification. Any time you ingest anything, stop and thank it for giving its life to sustain yours. Thank it and then thank the universe for providing for you. Don't overeat and don't waste food. Stay thankful and mindful at all times about the source of your food and what you will do to carry on its life force through you. All these sentient entities are giving their lives to sustain you, and you should feel both humbled by and grateful for this incredible responsibility. With this ingested life force, it now becomes your responsibility to *wake up* and spread grace and love on the planet.

Gardening

A key spiritual practice that can help you align with the energy of the Earth is gardening. There is an amazing communion between you and the planet when you grow your own food. If you have the ability to plant a garden at your home, go to the local nursery and buy an assortment of organic seeds or plants. If you don't have a yard, look into community gardens in your area or hydroponics. Many junior colleges have horticulture programs where you can study as well.

Growing our own produce is a very important practice that physically helps fuse our positive karma (action) with our sustained development. We actually enter into the loop of feeding ourselves and have the opportunity to *infuse* the soil, the crops, and the entire garden with our goodwill and healthy energy before we eat the food. In fact, we can program specific goals or medicinal "spells" into the food and tell ourselves that we will take on those characteristics once we ingest this food. It is an incredible method of entering into a live "biofeedback" loop with nature in how it intimately connects with us and sustains us. Don't worry if you can't produce enough in your house to feed your whole family (you might, though); just get involved in the ritual. Celebrating amazing tomatoes that you have grown is good enough for now.

Environmental Awareness

My teachers taught me that within fifteen feet of where we are standing (in a natural environment), nature usually provides a cure to whatever ails us. The incredible biodiversity on this planet is amazing, and it is important for us to partake of herbs and medicinal plants that grow close to where we live. Local botany is an important healing practice because it grounds us into the actual environment where we live. Get outside and learn about the local trees, plants, animals, and trends in the natural environment around you. Watch the birds and learn their calls. Become aware of the living, breathing biosphere in which you live.

It is so easy to take it all for granted as we race through our days. It is common to be wholly unaware of the energetic signature of the place where we dwell. Getting involved in local hikes and spending time learning about all the *life* around us is a powerful spiritual practice that is a sort of homecoming. *This* is where we evolved from. This is the environment of which we are an integral part. The human world and its crazy machinery is a bit too fast and insane compared to nature. Our return to our primordial home teaches us a great deal about ourselves and should be treated with the reverence it deserves.

Fasting

Another key component to the earth element purification is very much in line with the reverence practice mentioned above, and it is an age-old tradition found in most spiritual lineages. Fasting is incredibly important when done correctly, and it helps reinforce our understanding of nourishment and our relationship to the food chain here on the planet. Remember how we discussed the incredible power of food as a trance and how most of us go unconscious while we eat? Fasting is the key to unlocking that energy and unleashing the freedom trapped in that trance.

I recommend a water-only fast one day per week. This means, from morning to night, simply sipping room temperature water all day. Add a pinch of Himalayan sea salt here and there to balance electrolytes. There is no reason to overdo it, and it is important to not drink too much in one sitting (which will harm the kidneys). Make it a day where you can get away with exerting less energy and give yourself time for seated meditation or time in nature.

Now, I understand that this may be too much for many of you, but I am once again holding you to the gold standard in this book. If once a week is an undoable frequency for you right now, set aside one day a month and do it that way for now. Water fasting is an excellent way to detoxify the body and give the digestive system a break. It helps clear the mind and allows you to understand your relationship with food in a very deep way. It triggers something called *autophagy* which rids the body of defective cells.

Over the years, I've met a number of people who have fasted for religious convictions or to prove that they can, but they treated it like a monster that they had to overcome. Again, understand the nature of the reduction process and relax into a space of self-discovery and liberation with this. It is not self-torture and punishment. Over time, you will find that it is quite liberating and enjoyable. I know plenty of people who have fasted on water for twenty-one to forty days at a time. Of course, this is a bit more challenging and should only be done under the supervision of a qualified health-care professional.

It is also important to note that many people are hypoglycemic and/or have unhealthy variations in their blood sugar levels. For these people, I recommend a modified juice cleanse instead (until they can fix their problem and go to water). This cleanse consists of filtered, room-temperature water; freshly squeezed lemon or lime (use as much as you like); grade B maple syrup (approximately two tablespoons per liter of water); and organic green tea.

I have also recommended freshly squeezed juices for a number of patients, but the specific ingredients vary based on their condition. A good general combination is kale, celery, chard, apple, ginger, and carrot. Try to make 50 percent of the juice from the bitter ingredients (the first three in the list) and 50 percent from the flavorful ones (last three). Use only organic ingredients, and drink water in between all day to flush out the system. As mentioned, the ingredients will be a bit different for every person. Seek out a qualified health-care professional if you need some help deciding how to fast.

One thing that I like to add to all liquid fasts that I find quite helpful for spiritual development is a *vow of silence*. This works particularly well because we tend to have less energy to engage in interactions with people on these days, so we might as well do it all together! I find that most people spend the majority of their energy and zhi (or creative willpower) just spewing wasted energy out of their mouths all day. We literally create our reality with our thoughts and our words, so taking a regular break from speaking is an excellent way to fix the leak here.

PERSONAL JOURNEYS Fasting in Hawaii

I was heavily involved in my kung fu training while also taking twenty-four units at UCLA. I had a three-week break and needed the time to practice some of the techniques I had learned. Finals week commanded my attention, and I was committed to getting all A's, which I was able to do. But once finals were behind me, the time had come for a mini sabbatical.

I booked a three-week trip to Hawaii. I spent the first week with my family in Maui. I then flew to Kauai, where I spent one week alone in Waimea Canyon and another week on the Napali Coast. Waimea Canyon was completely empty, and I was the only person in there for the whole week. I found a nice campsite by the river and set up shop. My plan was to water fast for five days and go through a number of spiritual purification exercises. I didn't speak a word, and I allowed my body to cleanse and purify while I focused white light into my field. As I cleansed, I ran into a number of really uncomfortable feelings and memories; I felt like pulling out a number of times.

But the more I was able to let go and release, the easier it got, and the lighter I felt. At one point, I was able to follow a family of goats and stay within ten feet of them without their seeing me. I felt like I had blended in with the natural environment so well that they couldn't detect my odor or energetic signature. Although the first couple of days were rough, it got easier and more rewarding the further I went. By day five, I was ready to slowly get back into juices, as I would need more energy to hike several miles per day for the remainder of my trip. What was incredible to me was the amount of energy I felt during the fast. The more I cleaned up my energy field, the lighter and more energized I felt. My meditations were incredibly clear and comfortable, and several of the aches and pains I had been complaining about simply went away. When I was finally ready to eat solid food, I started with fruit. I picked a fresh mango off a tree, and I was in heaven. I was so thankful for that mango, and it tasted so delicious that I spent almost an hour eating it as slowly and mindfully as I could.

FIRE

Cleansing the fire element is very simple: cleanse fire with fire. One of the most ancient practices in the world is to use fire to purify one's energy and renew one's light; this is an excellent way to quickly "burn away" impurities and raise the vibration of the Light Body. Fire purification requires one simple ingredient: a nice healthy fire.

Now, we've all spent time in front of a fireplace or a campfire and have been captivated by its power and glow, but how often do we engage the *spirit of the fire* to cleanse our energy and purify our fields? A campfire is a three-dimensional reflection of the universal archetype of fire as an element and can be used for this purpose very well. Metaphorically, we can understand the nature of fire by examining its *gua*, or trigram (as shown in figure 10.1).

The upper and lower lines of the trigram represent the energy of yang, and the broken line in the middle represents the energy of yin. This image is in the binary code system of the *I Ching*, the Chinese book of oracles, which uses this system of straight and broken lines to describe all the phenomena in the whole universe.[1] Looking at a fire, we notice the abundant yang energy of the actual flames, which cannot exist without some form of *substance*. In this case, this substance would be the yin nature of the log.

This element becomes the microcosm of the metabolic processes that run in our bodies as well. We have our essence, which serves as the underlying basis for our material existence and which provides the substrate (the tissues that efficiently collect and organize burnable calories) for the metabolic processes of life to occur. This, in turn, kicks on the engines of the spirit to have a foundation from which to explore and learn.

FIRE RITUAL 1   FIRE CLEANSING

- Sit at a comfortable (and safe) distance from the fire and begin to breathe down to your lower dantien.

- Honor the fire by bowing to it; then allow its energy to permeate your field.

- State the following: "I give to you my impurities, my disharmonious energy, my sickness, and my sadness as fuel. Please purify these energies and cleanse my field by releasing the power in the darkness I've shared with you. Please continue to cleanse that which I cannot see in my shadow and help me return to the purity of my original state."

- Sit for as long as comfortable and allow the fire to cleanse your field.

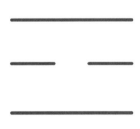

FIGURE 10.1   The Fire Trigram

- Thank the fire for the healing and sprinkle some frankincense or sage in it to purify the room or space.

FIRE RITUAL 2   THE TAOIST CANDLE MEDITATION

- Find a comfortable place in a dark room without any breeze; have a seat.

- Light a candle and place it about six to eight inches off the ground. Sit about two to three feet away from it.

- Place your hands on your knees, cupping the kneecaps, with thumb and index finger touching.

- Breathe in nose and out nose, with the tip of the tongue touching the roof of the mouth.

- Softly gaze at the blue part of the flame as you continue to breathe.

- Soften your gaze and try to avoid blinking your eyes.

- Allow the flame to really link up with your third eye and cleanse your spiritual vision.

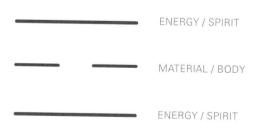

FIGURE 10.2   The Fire Trigram Breakdown

- Stay here as long as is comfortable and simply observe what you see (allow yourself to build up tolerance to this).

- When you are ready to close, pick up your hands, bring them into your chest (palms facing the flame) on the inhale, and then push your hands straight out on the exhale toward the flame. Mentally pull your consciousness *away* from the flame on the inhale and separate or cut your consciousness from the flame on the exhale. Do this for five breaths in nose and out mouth.

- Close your eyes and sit in silent meditation for a while.

METAL

Metal, the element of autumn, represents the declining cycle of nature. It is the energy of shedding off excess and giving back what is superfluous in our lives. A healthy tree sheds its leaves in the fall and even loses excess branches that are weak in order to be stronger the year after. It is important to understand that the excess that sheds from a tree gets mulched into the ground and becomes a powerful fertilizer that helps the tree's positive growth into the future. The compost also becomes the fuel and nutritional base for the seeds of its offspring into future generations. This is how life grows in nature, and it is exactly how we grow on all levels. Again, there is no distinction among mental, spiritual, emotional, and physical in reality; it's all One. However, coming from the perspective of polarity, we see the entire spectrum of this experience as distinct and different. Yin and yang help us *see* the unity in all things by creating a counterpoint perspective. When we understand this, we learn to see things correctly, of course.

Therefore, our spiritual purification practice for the metal element takes on the theme of release and renewal. The instructions for the practice that follow are in a more formalized standing form with some visualizations. Once you gain proficiency in the ritual (the same as with all the other concepts shared in this book), you can let this process work for you any time. But first, it is important to learn the essentials so that the key components are built into your practice. This particular exercise can be quite cathartic and intense at times, so make sure you are in a private, safe place. This is important for a couple of reasons. First of all, you will be in a very "exposed" position, so allow yourself the space to be raw and to molt. Second, a lot of chaotic energy will be spewing off you, so you want to make sure that it gets grounded into the earth and recycled. Some people who are very empathic can absorb vibrations easily, so make sure you take out your own trash.

The Vibratory State

Thanks to the pioneering work of Reverend John Davidson, professor Stanislav Grof, Leonard Orr, and Master Hong Liu, we have come to understand a profound method of release and renewal that encourages letting go in a very primordial way. Reverend Davidson (working intimately with the innovations of Alfred Korzybski) spoke of it very succinctly:

> The degree of strain in the nervous system which results from
> the conflict of language attempting to encompass feeling
> is the measure of "happiness and harmony." The degree of
> strain is determined, not through language, but through the
> "vibratory state," the body's reaction to language, . . . [and it]
> is in the vibratory state that original symbol selection can be
> demonstrated through resultant abreaction, and that "new
> symbols may be substituted for the old."[2]

In essence, language is an artificial human construct that cannot account for the energetic communication of personal feelings. Our subconscious mind understands what is going on, but the communication with our conscious mind gets processed through the imperfect language we have at our disposal. Not only do we lose so much in translation, we also use language to create "levels of abstraction" away from what Korzybski called the "original event," which further separates us from reality. The vibratory state is the disharmonious charge left in our system from the energy trapped in our shadows. This energy remains as we further reinforce it through our polarized thinking, which causes it to reverberate in our energy field until we reabsorb or discharge it. It is the reflection of the myriad vibratory frequencies we have trapped in our shadow.

All things want to grow, and all things grow toward the light. This is an important point to consider. The trapped energies of our shadow would naturally release and come to light if we were to leave things alone. In fact, if it were not for the *perpetual reinforcement and polarization* of our energy field, all things would self-correct naturally. We are the ones putting energy into this disarray, and we are the ones keeping it that way. We work at it day and night. We are exhausted by it. We spend all our energy fighting with reality and swimming upstream. The vibratory state is a perfectly natural reaction to energy trying to release. The more we allow what is trapped to be released through the acknowledgment of the original event, the more settled and less tumultuous our vibratory state becomes.

The vibratory state feels like (and oftentimes looks like) a mild trembling feeling. It can get to full convulsions with some energies or just a mild rocking or swinging back and forth with others. The practice of "shaking it out," described below, involves a passive scanning of the body and energy field for any disharmonious energies and then an "allowance" that frees these energies to finally express and release.

The critical mindset needed to perform this practice successfully is *acceptance*. Whatever comes up, simply acknowledge it, let it be, and allow it to express itself. Much like a small child who is being fussy and crying—ignoring it will not help, and neither will hostility. See what it wants. Let it be and allow it to move through your system in its own way until it expresses itself. Breathe into the area; the infusion of fresh energy with breath and the light of awareness will dislodge trapped energy and set it free.

Side note: All kinds of crazy stuff gets dislodged during this practice, and it is very common to look like we're almost having a seizure while in the vibratory state. Just breathe through it and let it be until it passes. Remember that it was the suppression of these energies that created the problem in the first place, so be accepting of whatever comes up and just let it be. That's all that would have happened at the original event anyhow had we not polarized, charged, encapsulated, and stored it so long ago! It would have come and gone like everything else; we were the ones who froze it in time and held onto it. This time, we've learned our lesson. Just let it be—whatever it is.

You can, if the motions get far too tumultuous, take a few attempts at releasing given energies. Chip away at it if you will. Oftentimes, you may feel like you are dying while in the vibratory state. That's not really the case, though you are dying *to this energy*. What is dying is the energetic "life-form" you've created around this subject. It's almost like a monster or a demon with a life of its own is kicking and screaming for its last breath. Stop feeding it your power and lovingly let it reabsorb into the universe. These are your falling leaves. Watch them as they are reabsorbed by the Earth and push up flowers. Do it with a smile on your face!

Preliminary Steps

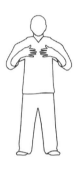

FIGURE 10.3
Post Position

- Go to a private room where you can be for a good twenty to forty minutes—preferably on the first floor of the building. Out in nature alone is ideal, although it may be impractical for most city dwellers.

- Stand in wu chi posture—feet shoulder-width apart and knees slightly bent.

- Put your hands into the post position, which looks like you are hugging a tree.

- Have the tip of the tongue touch the roof of the mouth and breathe in nose and out nose to the lower dantien.

- Allow your shoulders to relax and settle into the posture.

- Make the following statement to the Earth (in your mind or out loud): "Please absorb all of the energies that I am about to release to you. Let them be the food for tomorrow's flowers. Thank you."

- Remain in the same position. Begin to scan your body from head to toe and then back up for any discordant energies you may detect.

- It may take several passes to detect anything when you first start. When you sense one, simply acknowledge it and then allow your consciousness to "tune" into the vibration and let it resonate within you.

- Keep your breath focused on your lower dantien.

- Begin to allow your body to move with the energy (stay in the structure of the post position but move within this framework)—side to side, front to back, bouncing up and down, hands trembling. Do whatever naturally happens.

- Keep breathing down to your lower dantien and focus your attention on the vibratory state that you have just uncovered.

- Stay with this energy and keep breathing (and moving) with it until you feel like you have adequately discharged it.

- Again, allow any chaotic energy released to be absorbed into the Earth.

- Thank the energy for releasing and apologize to it for trapping it for so long.

- Move back into scanning for the next vibration if you still have an alchemical appetite. Repeat this sequence or move to the closing sequence.

You will find that the breathing becomes very erratic once you are in the vibratory state. You can choose to exhale out mouth as needed, but always return to your cyclic lower dantien breathing. The constant flow of breath and life force to this process is what brings in enough power to dislodge stuck energies. As you find the parts of the body that are holding trapped energy, you can often isolate precisely where the particular vibration is originating. Just keep breathing to *that specific area* and let the vibratory state continue to molt and unfold until it is done. Remember that these energies may have been trapped and reinforced for decades, so be patient with the process!

Closing Sequence

- Exhale out mouth and let the hands drop down to the sides.

- Inhale and circle the arms with palms up out to the sides and all the way to above your head (palms up); then exhale with palms down moving down in front of your body.

- Do this for three cycles, gathering energy up and smoothing the energy field on the way down.

- Give thanks to the Earth one more time and visualize, in your mind's eye, all the energy you discharged sinking into the ground and being absorbed. The further down it goes, the more flowers you see springing up at your feet all around you.

- Drink some water and relax for at least fifteen minutes. This would be a great time to go into some silent seated meditation to *see inside*. You'll be amazed at how clear the internal vision becomes when unhealthy energy is allowed to discharge.

To see a video sample of what this practice looks like, go to SoundsTrue. com/inner-alchemy/bonus. This is very powerful stuff, and it will change your life, so treat it with reverence and patience.

Side note: We do not live in a culture that accepts loss well; we love gains, but loss is "depressing" and very un-capitalistic. If you have a history of severe depression, psychosis, or any major mental illness, it is appropriate to proceed with caution in this process. Work hand-in-hand with your therapist to move through these techniques. In these cases, it is important to have someone there to deal with the fallout as things get shaken up. Remember, you are building the foundations of a strong oak tree from the dead leaves of yesterday. Two steps forward, one step back.

WATER

Water is the element of winter. It represents the energy of consolidation, nourishment, and regeneration. It is the rest and the gathering of qi and jing that allows us to fully express energy outwardly. It is the good night's sleep that gives us energy for the next day. It is the dark, peaceful silence that balances all the noise. Water makes up around 60 percent of the constituency of our bodies, and it is the "soup" in which all the processes of life work. In fact, water is the "currency" of life in many ways. It's our basis for growth and the driving force of all energy currents. There is a tremendous amount of energy traveling through water; this "liquid" energy flows throughout our bodies and is carried through all life-forms on the planet. Figure 10.4 shows the trigram for water.

Notice how this trigram is the inversion of the fire trigram. The trigram for water consists of a single yang bar between two yin bars. It conveys a soft external appearance that houses a tremendous yang power within. After all, it is water that carved the Grand Canyon, and it is water that carries that same power through every cell of our bodies.

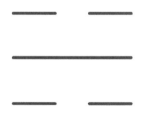

FIGURE 10.4   The Water Trigram

The spiritual purification practice for the water element involves a good amount of time in submersion in a clean source of water. Now, before you grab your swim trunks, chlorinated pools do not count, as chlorine can seep directly through the skin, creating a number of problems in our systems. Natural and unpolluted bodies of water are the best; in this particular practice, however, we will conduct our practice in a very convenient place—*the bathtub.*

Before we get into the instruction here, it is important to consider water quality in your home. Most of us live in urban environments where water is pumped and channeled from far away to get to our homes. Because of this, a number of chemicals are added to the water in order to ensure its safety from contamination. Millions of people die annually in lower-income countries because of polluted water, so it is quite a blessing to have clean water at our disposal. Modernity has its drawbacks, however, as separate health issues have arisen in concordance with the additives in our water. Because of this, it is important to not only have a filter for drinking water in the house but also to have a good shower filter. Our skin absorbs chemicals very effectively, and these chemicals create problems in our bodies, such as free radical damage and the weakening of gut flora colonies. Purchase a good filter for your shower (or whole house) and replace it as indicated. Use filtered water to fill the tub for this practice.

WATER PURIFICATION EXERCISE 1   SUBMERGED REJUVENATION

This practice is inspired by Leonard Orr's purification process, which I have found to be quite effective. Orr is the founder of rebirthing and has contributed much to this subject.[3]

- Fill your tub with filtered water and get it as hot as you can comfortably tolerate.

- You can add a pure source of sea salts or Epsom salts (preferable) if desired.

- Light a single candle within reach and then get into the tub. Submerge as much of your body as you can.

- Close your eyes and relax for a few minutes, allowing your body and mind to settle.

- *Circular breathing:* Begin a series of "connected breathing," which means connecting the inhale with the exhale without any pause in between. Do this for twenty continuous breaths. You can breathe in and out the nose here or out the mouth if you experience discomfort.

- After twenty breaths, relax and breathe down to the lower dantien for a number of breaths and observe what comes up.

- Just like the metal exercise, find whatever vibratory frequencies arise in your body and simply acknowledge them and allow them to be.

- Allow the water to purify and cleanse your energy body and absorb any chaotic qi.

- Once you feel like you have cleared a layer, move back into twenty more breaths of circular breathing. Repeat this cycle over and over for at least an hour.

- You will feel certain feelings of discomfort, and this will not always be fun. *Be* with those feelings and allow yourself to molt. The discomfort will pass, and you will then cleanse through to the next item in your shadow.

- When you finally sense you are done for this session, slowly drain the water and take a lukewarm to cold shower. This will seal the energy centers that you just worked on.

- Thank the water for helping you cleanse; return your breath to your lower dantien before exiting the shower.

This practice is incredibly cleansing and rejuvenating and can be done daily. That being said, there is always a trade-off between our personal needs and the state of the environment. Heating water for a bath requires a lot of energy, and a good amount of water is used. I tend to do this practice as a treat every now and again. If you have managed to work your way off the grid and have solar heating and can reclaim the water (no salt here!) for irrigation, then, by all means, do this practice more often. Natural hot springs are another excellent place to conduct this practice.

WATER PURIFICATION EXERCISE 2   BLESSING YOUR WATER

My grand master taught a special Taoist invocation using shen to "charge" a spell or idea into a glass of water. This water can then be given to a patient as medicine or taken for oneself. Since then, a good deal of excellent work has been done in the field of water research, and I feel that, with a healthy understanding of the principles taught in this book and the premise of Dr. Masaru Emoto's work on water, anybody can now practice this Taoist magic.[4]

The process is simple:

- Take a glass of filtered water and place it on a table in front of you.

- Put both your hands around the glass and simply breathe white light through your palms into the glass.

- Drop into your heart and say, "I love you," and "Thank you," to the water and hold that feeling in your heart.

- Allow that feeling to pass through your palms into the glass of water.

- Once the water is "blessed," you can add any other frequency you want to the glass. For example, penicillin, vitamin C, cough suppressant, caffeine—whatever you implant with your shen will be tuned into the water.

- Drink the water or give it to someone who needs it.

With practice, you will get better and better at this. I don't need to repeat the pioneering work of Dr. Emoto here, but it may suit you to read about it at some point. You will find that you can perform resonant tuning with any frequency pattern and do so quite effectively. The stating of "I love you" and "Thank you" miraculously *structures* the water into beautiful crystals, which, in turn, positively affects the alignment of water molecules in our bodies. This is also an excellent practice to do when in the bathtub. Simply turn your attention to the tub water and bless it before getting in. You can also implant a specific therapeutic intention into the tub water for your session.

CLINICAL ENCOUNTERS Blessing Our Water

I had a patient a few years back who had studied a variety of healing techniques and had put a lot of energy into learning how to heal. She displayed a variety of imbalanced fire element signs, and her entire demeanor pointed to this clearly. She had run into some health concerns while working as a busy executive and had decided to quit everything to study massage. She went from high-powered businesswoman to a crystal-wearing shamanic healer in the matter of two months. She had put away or given away all her possessions, and she was searching for answers everywhere.

Now, this all sounds good in theory, but what I found in front of me was a truly miserable person. She was running to the light but away from her life and her family. The flame of her heart fire had gone out of control, and she was making reckless decisions while compromising her lifelong relationships with a new, judgmental "spiritual" attitude. This wasn't liberation for her; it was just a rebellion.

After some discussion, I was able to convince her to try a balanced approach. I guided her to commune with the water element (which balances a fire disharmony) and gave her specific programming instructions for the water that she blessed and drank daily. It only took a month before she came to her senses. We were able to get her to take her keen business acumen and apply it to a new "green" business she had in mind. She went from spinning out of control and blowing through her life's savings to making great money while doing some real good for the world. She surrounded herself with good people and found a career that meant something. Her ailments had been cured, and she had her life back—all because we were able to balance her energy.

WOOD

The fifth and final element we will discuss in this section is the element of wood, which represents the emerging energy of springtime. It is the growth and the eternal will to live that we see sprouting up from all life. Wood energy carries with it enthusiasm and expansion. It is the emergent life force arising out of the restful winter—pushing to grow and thrive into the summer to come. This energy is easily detected and is almost contagious when "spring is in the air." It helps us fulfill our dreams and carries us forward with our ambitions. Although syncing up with the wood energy is easiest to do in the springtime, it is possible in any season just by going out into nature.

WOOD PURIFICATION EXERCISE 1 COMMUNING WITH A LEAF

Famous wilderness survival teacher and holder of the Apache tracking lineage, Tom Brown Jr. states that if you ever have a question about anything—*anything*—simply go meditate on a leaf and the answer will present itself.[5] I can get into fractal mathematics and attempt to explain why that makes sense with the new quantum science, but I'm not here to bridge that gap, and plenty of people can do that better than I can. Instead, I'm here to *show* you how to do this and open up the endless possibilities for you. The practice is as follows:

- Go out into a natural environment (if possible) and find a freshly sprouting leaf to meditate on (try not to pluck it off!).

- Sit comfortably and take ten breaths down to your lower dantien.

- Now, focus your attention on your heart center and then focus your eyes intently on the leaf (softly gaze at it without "bug eyes").

- Connect with the leaf through your heart and then continue to breathe in and out while focusing on the leaf.

- Really allow yourself to quiet the mind and *see* the leaf and all the intricacies in it while you continue to breathe and connect.

- Pose your question(s) to the leaf.

- Stay here for at least twenty minutes and breathe through any feelings of frustration, boredom, or general discomfort you may feel.

- When you are ready to close, return your breath and awareness to your lower dantien for another ten breaths.

- Wish the leaf well and bow to it before getting up.

You want to ideally find a young healthy leaf to practice this on, but at the end of the day, any leaf will do. Once you are able to communicate with the sentience of the leaf and after the language of the underlying life force speaks to you, the fun really starts. Remember: all of life is emerging through the same universal fractal pattern, so any part of the whole contains all the information of the universe (past, present, and future). The leaf is simply a budding snapshot of that pattern, which places it right in your face. Actually, that pattern is always right in your face, all the time! Once you bite into the mystery of mysteries, you'll realize why the great masters are always laughing.

WOOD PURIFICATION EXERCISE 2   RANDOM ACTS OF KINDNESS

The spiritual attribute of the wood element is that of benevolence, which acts as a counterweight to the disharmony expressed in anger, frustration, and depression. The wood element is considered the "general" of our systems. It takes the heart's desires and carries them throughout the body. Subsequently, the wood element is our body's "doer"—the element that gets things done. So, if we examine the types of mental or emotional pathologies that emerge with a disharmonious wood element, we see problems with action. Anger is aggressive action energy coming as a response to something we have an aversion to. Frustration is a sense of pent-up energy from action that didn't quite manifest in the desired result. Depression is the energy of giving up on action that has been frustrated. They are all tied into how we move toward our desires or away from things we can't tolerate. Most people in the West have wood element pathologies because they feel like they always have to "do something" to fix things or change reality to their liking. Remember the Lucifer Experiment from chapter 2?

The ancient Taoist teachings tell us that once we come back to balance and harmony with the Tao, all action becomes spontaneously inspired and driven from the power within versus mental reactions to emotional charge. This is a wonderful place to be and to cultivate, but we first need to bridge that gap by taking the edge off this deep-seated pathology to do something. So, here we are again: finding a problem and attempting to *do something* about it! We are fighting imbalanced action with more imbalanced action.

The nature of the next exercise is very similar to the mental practice meditation discussed earlier. That practice asked us to observe any and all action in our mind and simply *stop doing it*. The only action acceptable in that practice is asking the question: "What am I doing right now?" and then stopping whatever mess we find ourselves in and calmly returning to a state of inaction.

In this next practice, we are going to follow that same line, but instead of practicing *inaction*, we are going to practice the only karmically healthy form of action out there: *benevolence*. This means performing good deeds for the benefit of *all life*.

PERSONAL JOURNEYS **Letting Go of Attachments**

While in India, I purchased a *mala* prayer bead necklace, and I took it along with me wherever I went. Every great master I encountered and studied with, including the Dalai Lama and Karmapa Lama, blessed it for me. These particular prayer beads are built with a counting system wherein you slide a disc to one side for every time you say a prayer. You slide another one over for every hundred. There was another counter that I slid over for every time I finished ten sets of one hundred, which made a thousand. I was told I needed to say the Tibetan prayer *Om mani padme hum* ("hail to the jewel of the lotus") into this mala *ten thousand times* to activate it. It took dozens of bus rides and hundreds of hours of patiently praying into this thing for over six months until I had finally reached ten thousand. This *relic* was the single most valuable thing I possessed, and I was so proud to have prayed into it and have it been blessed by so many saints. I guarded it with my life and never took it off.

There I was, reveling in the beauty of my new toy when my inner voice came in loud and clear. I was instructed to give it to a friend of mine back in Los Angeles! I tried to pretend I didn't hear it, but the feeling was unavoidable. When I returned to the States, I simply handed it over to this person as a souvenir and carried on about my business. I thought about it often and occasionally still do. It was like Bilbo Baggins (*The Lord of the Rings*) giving away his *precious* ring of power to Frodo. It was a powerful lesson in nonattachment, and it has taught me much about externalizing spirituality. It was the act of doing the prayers that meant everything. The material object . . . well, be careful, because that was a shiny trap!

Part of the pathology of our Western Creation myth is that we should do good deeds for other *humans* and that we may do so at the expense of the environment, which God has told us is under our dominion anyhow. Not anymore! Make sure your definition of doing good deeds includes all life, all sentient beings, anything you see or don't see, *all that exists*. We are all One and part of the same life force, so excluding *anything* creates polarity and separation in the very fabric of the universe. Please don't do that!

The practice is a simple one: perform five random good deeds every day. Do more if you can, but aim for a minimum of five. Such acts could range from helping a person in need to picking up trash on the beach when you see it. Maybe it is giving a compliment to a stranger who looks like they need it. You decide. The quickest way to heal a wood element pathology is to start inundating the world with genuine good deeds. If you must do something, at least do good! It makes the world a better place and helps us get out of our narcissism.

On that point, I'd like to emphasize the importance of anonymity in this work (as much as is possible). We are not performing these acts for the cultural accolades we receive but just *because*. Our egos would love to take credit for these actions, though, just as our egos would love to make us the hero, the saviors of humanity, the martyrs, and the saints. Drop it! Be anonymous and simply do good deeds without any conditions or strings attached. Let your higher self perform the good deed, not your ego.

WOOD PURIFICATION EXERCISE 3   CLEANSING ANGER

As mentioned earlier, it is pent up anger that leads to frustration. We become depressed when we detach and don't do anything about it, and we become full of rage when we let it swell up for too long inside. The Taoist perspective on this is to release or discharge repressed emotional energy in a controlled and meaningful fashion. I am always surprised at how much repressed anger I see in people in our society. People are overflowing with it. For me, I have spent a good deal of time in the martial arts, where we have an organized and effective platform to work out aggression. Some of the nicest people I have met are seasoned martial artists who have come full circle and found inner peace through a deep understanding of their anger and pent-up frustrations. I also meet "spiritual" teachers who look like they are about to explode.

The conscious act of moving anger through us and allowing it to express in a controlled setting is both liberating and empowering. Holding onto anger is like having a gong go off in our head and being unable to do anything about it. It will eventually drive us to kick in a wall. That's why I highly recommend an organized martial arts discipline if possible. If not, a great way to work out some aggression is to put on some gloves and lay into a punching bag or a pillow. Do it somewhere in a safe environment and really allow yourself to get deeply into the field of the anger as you simply open up the floodgates and let it move through you. Remember, all energies want to move and express naturally. Allow the anger to release and move through you and out into the punching bag, as hanging onto it gives it more charge, and it will eventually consume you. Once you are done (or exhausted), sit in silent meditation and visualize a green light around your body. Bring your attention back into your lower dantien and notice what has changed inside. Now, this process is an excellent way to let off the pressure that has built up over the years. It may take several attempts to feel clear of these pent-up feelings, so stay with it. But remember, this practice does not *fix* the problem.

The problem with anger is usually the swallowing of our words when a boundary is violated. Sometimes it is appropriate to be upset about a certain thing. For instance, if an elderly woman is trying to cross the street and no cars are stopping for her at the crosswalk, it is perfectly appropriate to get out there and help her cross while sharply signaling the violators to stop. Standing up for what is right and just is critical; it is usually when we swallow our words and keep them inside that they turn into anger and frustration. When you speak your truth and are honest and raw in life, there is less to swallow. When boundaries are crossed, we feel violated. If that keeps happening to you, work on strengthening your boundaries. Do this with the relationships in your life. Do this by strengthening your wei qi using the qi gong exercises described earlier.

Anger is just another emotion, and it has received a very negative connotation in our culture because we judge it as "bad." What is truly "bad," however, is our reluctance to be real and raw in the moment. We feel like we are not being good people when we feel angry, so we hide it. We bottle it up and store it for years; then, one day, we snap at our spouse for something silly they do, and it blows up into an explosion of dramatic proportions. When we speak our truth in the moment and let people know that a certain action, comment, or behavior bothers us *when we first encounter it*, we help establish healthy boundaries and prevent the creation of yet another internal demon.

This concludes part II of this book. Practice what you've learned and keep your focus on using these techniques to "subtract" or to simplify your life and to clear blockages in your field. You will soon begin to feel more energy and clarity available to you on a day-to-day basis. This energy is nothing new; it's always been there, but most of us are too busy creating that mess we call our lives to actually *feel* all that power moving through us.

In part III, we will explore what we can now do with this information and get into the implications of what that means for our personal growth and development. We'll look directly into the light at the end of this tunnel and get our bearings straight. Our sleepy trances would like to convince us that we're not worthy or that this course of action is not for us. But *we now know better*! We are going to plot a course and boldly push through and claim our birthright!

PART III

COMING HOME

11

THE PREDATORY UNIVERSE

The only freedom warriors have is to behave impeccably.
Not only is impeccability freedom;
it is the only way to straighten out the human form.

CARLOS CASTANEDA, *The Second Ring of Power*

Now that we have laid the groundwork and learned the collective practice that is going to clean our energy field, it is time to look directly into the face of the monster and gain some appreciation for the magnitude of the problem as it relates to us and the world in which we live. We have developed an understanding of how we interface with reality and how we leak energy into our shadows through our reactions. We have learned that this is what creates the trance mentality, which makes us walk around like zombies, 90 percent asleep and constantly suffering on all levels. It is this leaking of our energy that opens us up to the "black market" of energy exchange. This is the predatory reality that has us feeding off each other and allows other entities to live off us all.

Recall from chapter 6 that we have the vertical "spiritual" axis of fire and water (figure 6.1). This axis fuses attention and intention with the central intellect that serves as the basis of our major alchemical work. We also have the horizontal "soul" axis of wood and metal through which the intellect tries to process the rising and falling circumstances of our lives (figure 6.2). It is through this horizontal axis that the intellect develops the ego, which in turn serves as a fortified identity to help us deal with day-to-day life. This is also from where we leak a great deal of our energy through our aversions and cravings. It is from within this horizontal axis that we "bleed" into our shadows. Through this process, we pump energy into the opposite polarity of whatever makes us uncomfortable, while we also reinforce beliefs and characteristics in our ego that help "protect" us from the way we feel about these things. Over time, we create clusters or families of these reactions that thematically join and form our fear-inspired beliefs and subconscious behaviors. These behaviors are subconscious by nature because they come from our shadows—the light of conscious awareness doesn't see them, so they go unchecked. We, in turn, walk around in a trance most of the time. *Then, we run into each other.*

It's bad enough having one zombie around, but what happens when there are more? What if almost *everyone* is asleep? Well, just take a look around you. In reality, we are all truly One, and the perception of separation is part of our ignorant sleep; therefore, we all affect and exchange with each other all of the time. We have a permanent, spiritual flu that keeps being endlessly passed from one person to another because everyone is unaware of the cure. The same way a thematic series of thought aversions bundle together to create a subconscious belief in own your shadow is how it happens within the shadows of others. In fact, we tend to attract like-minded people into our fields for good reason.

Think about this example: When he was a young child, John had a single bad experience with a schoolmate who happened to be black. That experience created a specific charge of aversion in him against that particular boy. Then he saw that boy hanging out with a couple other black boys, so he extended his judgment against "those boys." He avoided them in the halls and tried not to sit by them at lunch. He then told his friend about this dislike, because every time he saw any of that group of boys, he felt uncomfortable. His friend said that his father told him to watch out for black people because they steal. John couldn't help but feel vindicated. The energy in his shadow, which had already taken life from his own aversions before, had now taken on a new belief system—that black people steal. This happened easily because the original charge remained unexamined; therefore, the subsequent addition went straight through without any conscious rationale. John and his friend then found further vindication in their belief by talking to a few other boys, and suddenly they had all created a hostile environment for the black boys—who couldn't even figure out why this was all going on.

Twenty years later, John moves into a "safe" neighborhood where they don't let "those" people in, and he talks about how inner-city people are all lazy and that we need more prisons to contain "them." Funny enough, somehow he has lumped Arabs, Mexican immigrants, and a few other races of people into his belief system over the years. "These people are not to be trusted. . . *I'm buying a gun.*"

This example can go on and on because every time John has an aversion to anything that pulls up the "race" theme, it gets filed into this folder and feeds the monster in his shadow. He develops a huge array of subconscious behaviors that he simply accepts as self-evident truths, but he has no real rational or conscious foundation for any of it. Does this guy sound familiar?

The fact of the matter is that we're all involved in this game all the time, unless and until we wake up and understand how it functions within us. We do it with everything. We recruit people who share our likes or dislikes into our lives subconsciously, and we help each other reinforce these beliefs through "mob mentality."

Puppeteers

There are the billions of people walking around this planet who are completely ignorant of their behaviors, and then there are those who have finally discovered the cure and woken up, but merely to a certain degree. There are only two ways to go once we start arising from the human trance: either we see the plight of your fellow humans and feel *compassion*, committing our life to somehow helping them and making the world a better place, *or* we see the inherent weakness in their vulnerable state and understand that we have *leverage over them*.

The first category of people is interested in your own further awakening and embracing of the universal love of the life force, channeling it through themselves to help you see clearly—even if it might only be for a moment. These are the great saints and teachers who have come and gone. They are also the millions of people who are committed to helping humanity to some degree and on some level. These people don't have to be fully awakened to have their heart in the right place. Sadly, the great majority of them still carry a polarized charge in their shadows. Because of the nature of the shadow, these things are unconscious by definition, and it often leaves this whole class of people open to being manipulated and coerced.

The other category is that group of people who can (to varying degrees) see through the behaviors of others and who understand *how* to invoke archetypal arguments and "mob mentality" in order to leverage people into fulfilling their own desires. There are people who are very skilled in the esoteric arts who are quite active in this realm, but they are not alone. We all do it unconsciously. Like a good judo fighter, we learn to see weakness in each other through our subconscious processes. We throw and get thrown—always engaged in some wrestling match all the time. Unfortunately, those who get quite good at this are often the ones who are the most "successful" in worldly affairs. Because they are the ones who comprehend and execute this manipulation the best, they have leveraged all of society to see things their way.

If you create a monetary system and lend it to governments of the world and if that "money" is considered the currency of freedom, power, abundance, and value in our culture, then he with the most is at the top. Who is the one with the most? How about the one who created the game and who issues the money in the first place? A number of individuals have gotten this game down and have billions of people globally buying into their way of living life. Because people are completely asleep, they can't even question things—"It's just how things are." This system works all the way down as well. When a car dealer sees a middle-aged guy on his lot staring at a red sports car, he knows the exact angle to leverage this guy into getting his money. *Let's see . . . wants to feel desirable again . . . has some money . . . wants to impress girls . . . is feeling insecure.* Easy—convince him that this car will make him feel better and fulfill his myriad desires.

The advertising industry is essentially built on the exploitation of human emotions: fears, desires, insecurities, and beliefs. *You have to buy this home alarm system because the world is not safe, and someone is going to get you!* Because we don't have conscious awareness of what is going on within ourselves, many people all around us have learned to feed off the energy in our shadows and get what *they* want. In fact, the virtual "black market" of energy is where most people go to get their daily fix. The great majority of their conscious energy has been ripped off, so they need to get into the game and get more. Either you become a predator, or you lock yourself up with depression and anxiety and avoid people and the "rat race." Because we have lost so much of our personal power to our shadows, we feel tired and drained. Because we need to keep functioning in our day-to-day jobs and lives, we need to get the lost energy from somewhere. So we drink stimulants and start to drain energy from each other. We have become a culture of vampires sucking life force from wherever we can every day, just to get by.

Money and Sex

Money and sex are two of the biggest hang-ups for people in our culture when it comes to leaking vital energy. They hold pivotal spots in people's consciousness and carry deep-seated anxiety and fear-inspired beliefs, which lead to harmful behaviors. Let's start with money.

We live in a culture where there has been a strange juxtaposition of beliefs on the subject of money. The religious heritage of many people has inserted a deep-seated "money is evil" program that is always running in the background. Along with this comes thoughts like, *Rich people all gain their wealth unethically*, or *I don't want money to corrupt me.* This type of programming gets superimposed on the reality of the economic system in which we live. In the United States, money talks. Commercials are constantly prodding us to buy new products or change our look in order to be desirable. We have forces pulling on us from all sides trying to get us to spend our hard-earned cash, and, in the end, most of us do. *I need this new car because I deserve it*, and *This purse is so outdated, so I need a new one,* are common types of thoughts. These things cost money, and we are happy to pay or finance our way into getting the stuff that we desire. *Fine.* Make money and buy what you desire.

The problem is that most Americans have learned from their government and are too happy to borrow and get into deficit spending.

Everyone is stressed about money, and the subject occupies way too much of our daily mental energy. In order to be free of this pathology, we really need to balance our personal budgets and be more mindful about our expenditures. There is nothing inherently wrong or evil with money; it is our *relationship* with money that creates profound stress and anxiety in our daily lives.

Sex, on the other hand, is a broad and sensitive subject that needs to be teased out here a bit. Sex sells. It is the driving force behind so much of our culture and our consumption-based economy; it is literally everywhere. Makeup, clothing, cars, music . . . you name it—there's some aspect of sales that ties in sex. Why? Sex is the fundamental energy that drives our species. Sex is our connection to our immortality and all our life force. It defines who we are, and our egos are leveraged by it. Our "sex appeal" is really important to us because it ties into some deep primitive mammalian genes. People are so lost in their mental sexual meanderings that they can be leveraged by people who understand what's going on.

The solution to this pathology is actually quite easy: learn Tantra. Tantra is the ancient spiritual art of personal cultivation that teaches us to harness, control, and work with our sexual energy. The aim is to raise and refine this energy to the spiritual centers of the brain and to learn to harness and control this force. This is the path to an ultimate source of power and realization that cannot even be described. The leaking of sexual energy is equal to spiritual suicide in the Tantric sense. This energy must be understood, cultivated, and, more important, celebrated once we realize the beauty and magnitude of it.

Vampires and Demons

It's not hard to create an artificial demon. Here's an excerpt from the Western Hermetic tradition:

> How are demons engendered? As with all generation, that of demons is the result of the cooperation of the male principle and the female principle, i.e., the *will* and the *imagination*, in the case of generation through the psychic life of an individual. A desire that is perverse or contrary

to nature, followed by the corresponding imagination, together constitute the act of generation of a demon.[1]

Let's look at this excerpt closely and piece it together in the language we have learned in this book.

- A desire that is perverse or contrary to nature is a reaction to a thought or emotion that reflects an aversion or a craving. In essence, nature unfolds for us in a particular way, and our reaction results in a desire "away" from this flow.

- The male and female principles are the *will*, which is the zhi housed in our kidneys (female, water, yin), and the *imagination*, which is the attention or shen housed in the heart (male, fire, yang).

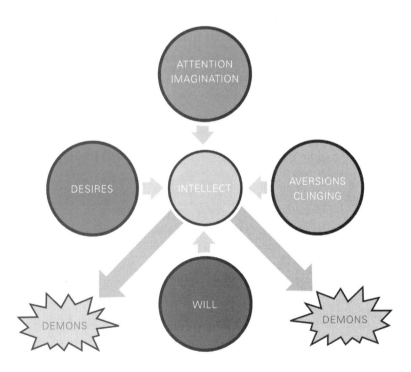

FIGURE 11.1   How We Create Demons

- We have a desire or reaction on the horizontal axis, and we use the vertical axis to create in accordance with this. Therefore, when we have an unnatural desire, we use our creative principle to create an artificial demon.

This is exactly what we have been talking about since the beginning of this book, but I have avoided using the aggressive nomenclature until now. The energy we pump into our shadows that breathes "life" into our aversions and cravings actually creates artificial demons that take on a life of their own and begin to influence our mind and activities. This mechanism is illustrated in figure 11.1.

In this faulty model, our mind and emotions have an abreaction to whatever reality is presenting, and, using our creative faculty, we polarize the energy and literally breathe life into demons we have created that live in our shadows. These demons then influence our thoughts and create similar situations for us in life that draw us into similar abreactions, which, in turn, continue to feed these demons. This is what is called an *internal possession* in Taoism. The way we conduct an exorcism in this situation is exactly how we have been doing it all along in this book.

- We acknowledge the behavior and bring the light of consciousness to it.

- We stop engaging in our habitual pattern of reinforcement through aversions and cravings.

- We drop into our heart center and forgive the person, situation, or thing that is causing our internal reaction.

- We "watch" as the energy deflates and dissipates while we hold it in love and withdraw the power we have put into its opposite polarity.

- We search our consciousness for similar energies or demons and perform the same process.

Essentially, we get in and exorcize our own internal demons, because if we don't, they will keep drawing us into unhealthy unconscious behavior until our last moment in our earthly bodies. In fact, once our demons have enough power in our shadows, they constantly drain us of our vitality. This, however, starts to diminish their source of energy, so that one of three things happens:

- We continue to get drained and, at a certain point, become devoid of essential vitality. Our ying (nutritive) qi becomes compromised, and we get ill and eventually die unless an intervention is sought.

- We learn to "import" energy from the outside world, at first through stimulants and drugs—anything to squeeze more energy out of our present situation. Eventually, we learn to take energy from others, and then we become vampires (unconsciously) as our internal demons find ways of having other people give us their power.

- We gain awareness of this cancerous cycle and stop feeding our demons. They kick and scream for a short time and then wither and die off. The more qi gong we practice and mental awareness we have, the easier we are able to clear ourselves of these parasites.

Unfortunately, there are a lot of people in the first two categories listed above and precious few in the third. Now that you are this far into this book, it is your responsibility to step up and clear your parasites. By bringing vitality and awareness to your energy field, you will dispel all your own internal demons and then become very aware of the vampirical/predatory nature of the world around you. You can then illuminate this behavior and help the people around you snap out of it. With enough people waking up, the cycle is broken, and humanity is freed from this trance.

Human Transference

Human transference is the most common form of possession out there. It is rampant in the United States and gets carried through from generation to generation. We see it in sexual predators and pedophiles, as well as in those with addictions and in perpetrators of domestic violence. It occurs when the demons are so empowered that they draw someone into an action that they would not otherwise do. Many of these people often claim that "something came over me" or "I just couldn't stop myself, even when I knew better." This is a classic example of the shadow having more energy than the conscious part of the energy field; this is when we are no longer in control, and, frankly, there's trouble. When this happens, a person who has left their psyche and their field "unchecked" for years *infects* another person (or group of people) through their actions. For example, we know that the majority of sexual predators were molested in their past. Like a mental virus, it carries on from the perpetrator to the recipient/victim and plants the seeds for further growth. If the victim does not heal the trauma and forgive the situation, then they harbor this "infection" in their own shadow. When they become weakened at some point, they may find themselves expressing this demon—much to their own surprise.

We do this with everything. We transfer belief systems and ideas into each other's subconscious minds because we are unaware of their existence. (Again, this is how advertising and political campaigns work; in fact, these two professions have this down to a science.) Many of us are unaware of our demons and have unexamined shadows; when we are in a "sleepy moment," our shadow is able to overpower our conscious actions, which allows these demons to express themselves. Just like a virus, they have taken on a life of their own, and they feed off our energy; to survive, they must *infect* the next person they come in contact with. The more culturally appealing these demons might be, the quicker they can spread into more host bodies. They have been called *memes* in popular literature, and there is a good deal of discussion arising on the subject; for example, look to the 1996 work *Virus of the Mind*, by Richard Brodie, for a more detailed account. We are unconscious to this transference and become the willing agents of this process through our ignorance.

External Demons

We have spoken of people manipulating each other for personal gains and of internal demons taking on charge and manipulating behavior for their own survival and proliferation. Now, we must talk about a more insidious energy—external entities that are disembodied.

Many of the entities that fall into this category are former humans that, for one reason or another, were "trapped" in our dimension after losing their bodies. Either they had something that held them back from willingly leaving, or, more frequently, their death was so jarring or quick that they don't believe they are truly dead. These are often ghosts of relatives that are reported in houses around the world. There are thousands of these stories all over, and anybody who has actually encountered one of these entities will not be convinced by anyone who says that they don't exist. These entities are actually relatively easy to deal with; just like the internal demons, they need a source of energy to live off for survival. If we stop feeding them, they lose their power and must move along. Now, very much like the feeding of our internal shadow energies, we feed these entities through our minds and our emotions.

Having a human body is quite special, and it is the ultimate source of infinite power, once we know how to tap into it properly. Disembodied entities can latch onto us or our ideas and live off them for long periods. Haunted houses are a good example because the entity oftentimes inspires fear, which is a powerful, raw energy in the people around the house. The more people who acknowledge that the house is haunted and that this entity exists, the more energy is available to it. Dead relatives also will provoke such strong emotions because they have to stoke the fire of their own memory in their living loved ones in order to "drink" the energy that is given off from the ensuing grief or fond feelings aroused. It is important to remember that most of these entities do not want to be trapped here and that we can release them by acknowledging what they are and then creating a portal for them to return back to the Source. These entities have no power outside of the power we give them unconsciously. And please remember, *they are us*. Love them and give them the space to find their way back home.

Insidious Demons

There are also more insidious energies out there that come from other planets or dimensions or that are created by dark masters here on this planet. They were called *archons* by the early Gnostics or *jen* by the Persians, and they have been classified into many subclasses by various cultures around the world. In fact, every culture somehow alludes to them in some way. These entities often have far more dangerous intentions and are to be avoided at all costs. All of these entities feed off the energy of fear the easiest, so it is critical for us to stay in our hearts and bring the energy of love and grace into the room. Nineteenth-century French poet, Charles Baudelaire's maxim applies today: "The finest trick of the devil is to persuade you that he does not exist."[2]

There is very special training that goes into Taoist exorcisms, which is beyond the scope of this book. It can be very easy to try to blame some outside agency/energy for the way we feel or possibly blame someone closer to home—perhaps we believe that Mom and Dad are the culprits. However, this blame game is not the way to fix anything! Again, we are responsible for our own awareness, and we are the only ones capable of cleansing our energy field. The more we reclaim our own power back and return to our center, the less our internal demons have leverage over us, which means the less we are in trance and the more we will be able to move toward positive energies and opportunities in our lives. When we wake up to our true potential, no demon, internal or external, will be able to influence us or get in our way ever again.

Farmers vs. Hunters

Taking into account all of this predatory activity and the nature of our horizontal leaching off of one another, it becomes important to hold a new frame of mind when encountering people and engaging in the outside world. We are surrounded by millions and millions of what the Buddhists call "hungry ghosts." They are devoid of their own power and are seeking to partake of some of yours in order to get through their day. They are lost to their internal demons and are trying to enroll you in their dramas. They are being led by the puppeteers into voting and buying the way they are told, and they are also after your money. But wait. They are you, and you are they!

Before we get into a reactive polarized "us versus them" mentality, let's realize that these are our brothers and sisters and that we are all in this mess together. The good news about waking up is that it can happen rather quickly and that it is the *birthright* of every human being on this planet. So, before we start to build walls around us and freak out about vampires and zombies attacking at the gates, let's gather ourselves and get into the work.

When I was younger and had just created my integrated medical group, there was a great deal to learn and lots of different models to emulate. I hired a business consultant whose "vibe" I liked (and he also came well recommended), and we got to setting up systems so that we could efficiently help as many people as possible. One thing that he taught me early on was that most business people in the United States act like hunters nowadays. They are out to pull down their daily feast, thinking that tomorrow is a new day with new quotas. Their lives are filled with lots of excitement and lots of stress—always trying a new angle to get the sale and win people over. Farmers, on the contrary, take the time to develop their relationships (crops) and to water and nourish them. At first, things start off slowly, but then, the yields get greater and greater, and the farmer ends up with an abundance of crops that keep rolling in. In regard to a health-care practice, this farming attitude meant creating a "family practice" environment where we cultivate our relationships with people and establish rapport and trust for years to come. In the perspective of the conversation at hand, being a farmer means moving out of the predatory frenzy of the horizontal axis and literally farming our energy field—tilling the soil and pulling weeds constantly.

Now that we have conducted a semantic "full circle," let's take a moment to examine the words we are using in this practice: *energy field*. A field denotes a space that is fertile and is to be cultivated. The field is yin in nature, taking seeds (yang) and nurturing them to grow. It is the space where water and nutrients mix to hold the space for life-forms to grow and evolve when activated by sunlight. The healthier the field, the better the yield. However, some fields are more fertile than others because they are endowed with rich nutrients from a volcano or are in a river delta where water and silt are abundant. This is much like our body. Some of us are born with strong jing/essence and have a lot to work with, while others, like a barren desert, have more challenges to keep things growing. Either way, after a number of seasons, if there is abuse or neglect from the farmer, the field starts to get compromised and cannot support the life and growth it used to. The soil needs to be turned, and weeds need to be extracted. It takes a good amount of work to keep a field healthy, but the rewards are immeasurable. This is exactly the same with our body.

Our energy fields are a direct reflection of the state of health of the jing, qi, and shen. If the energy is flowing smoothly and the diet and lifestyle are healthy, then there is a strong energy field, and the Light Body begins to take hold. If there is a disconnect in any of these parameters and if we are being drained by ignorance, then our shadow demons become fast-growing weeds in our fields. The crops we choose to grow are the dreams and aspirations of our heart, but the ones we end up growing are a result of the noise in the shadow. All it takes is fear-inspired desire or the charging of an aversion, and there we have it: another weed sprouts. The more we water that weed with our leaky energy, the more of our field we lose, and the more of a mess we have to deal with.

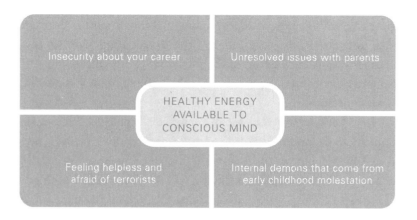

FIGURE 11.2   Unhealthy Energy Field

In a flat, unhealthy energy field, as shown in figure 11.2, we have very little of our total energy available to us when the energies of the shadow are still being fed. Once we begin the Great Work of Tao and start to tend to our fields daily, we can pull the energy out of the unconscious shadow processes and allow it to nurture our healthy core.

As we gather more and more personal power back within our conscious grasp, we are able to *use* more of it to pull weeds and exorcise our demons. We, at this point, are feeling better and better about ourselves and have the energy and vitality to address issues and meet life head on. With our continued practice of qi gong and the mental, emotional, and spiritual practices we have learned here, we continue to refine and clean until the Great Tao is finally in the driver's seat, instead of all the noise. The "I" that was created by the ego as a defense mechanism gets softened and dissipates in charge, and we surrender ourselves to the joyful manifestation of reality as it unfolds in front of us—and we watch ourselves unfold with it.

At this point in the book, we have sufficiently defined the "problems." From the next chapter on, it is time to really put things together and delve into the essence and meaning of this esoteric practice. It is time to really grasp the light at the end of the tunnel and to set our sights for *nothing short* of complete enlightenment and the full activation of our Light Body.

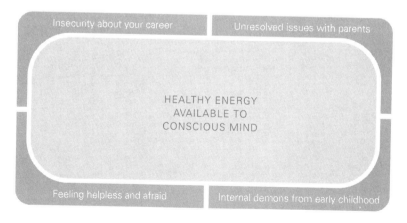

FIGURE 11.3   Healthy Energy Field

12

THE TAO OF MANIFESTATION

Turning the light around is the secret of dissolving darkness
and controlling the lower soul. There is no exercise to restore
the creative, only the secret of turning the light around.
The light itself is *the creative*; to turn it around is to restore it.

LÜ TUNG PIN, *The Secret of the Golden Flower* (translated by Thomas Cleary)

Throughout this book, we have spent a good deal of time examining what happens as a consequence of our ignorance of the natural processes around us. We have learned about how we channel energy into creating internal demons in our shadows and how these demons, in turn, begin to control and influence our behaviors. We have also seen how this phenomenon leads to a culture of vampirism, codependency, and mind control. As a result, we see how suffering creates a rift in our awareness of nature and how this fundamental split sends us down a dark and sleepy path toward further ignorance and deterioration. In short, we have circled around the problem, and now it is time to focus on the correction.

Up to this point, we have studied the energetic, mental, emotional, physical, and spiritual exercises that are designed to bring balance to our energy and to help increase the flow of vitality in our field. Now we must take control of the very system that has gotten us into so much trouble: it is time to program our subconscious mind and restore the powerful "trinity" that allows us to be masters of our own universe.

We have examined the mental and emotional aspects of our afflic-
tion, as these are the processes that channel our vitality into the shadow.
We have learned that it is by the very nature of this subconscious programming that we embed energies into the shadow that then take on a
life of their own. These "demons," if you will, suck our vital force and
live off our energy field like parasites. *It is the lack of clarity and conscious communication between our conscious mind and our subconscious
mind that allows this to be possible.* It is this fundamental disconnect
that lets there be a leak in the first place. Once we begin the process of
pulling weeds from our energy field, however, we become clearer and
clearer, reclaiming more and more of our conscious awareness.

The major function of the Taoist alchemical tradition is to turn the light
of awareness *inward* so that we can examine ourselves. Our alchemical

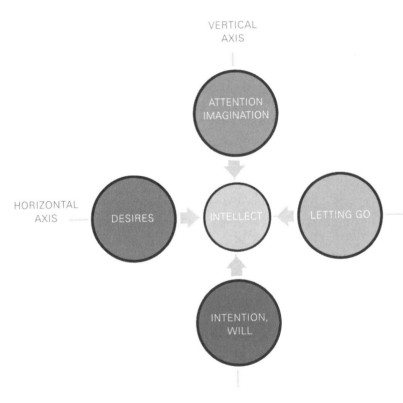

FIGURE 12.1   The Five Element Spirit/Soul Axis

work creates the environment for us to then take control of the seeds we plant and have more of an active role in the unfolding of our life.

When we consider the five element spirit/soul axis (figure 12.1), we see that the horizontal axis and the vertical axis all meet and communicate at the central level of the intellect (yi). This is the birthplace of the ego, where we create coping mechanisms for the energies we feel along the horizontal axis.

This is what we call our self-consciousness. It is the conscious aspect of our self-understanding, and it is the self-aware aspect of our energy field. This level of consciousness sits balanced between the poles of superconsciousness (the yang heaven aspect) and subconsciousness (the yin earth aspect), as shown in figure 12.2.

Just like when the polarization of the Tao created a spectrum between the extremes of yin and yang in every particular thing and concept, we can view our consciousness under the same light. We can say that the superconscious yang awareness is associated with heaven and the subconscious yin awareness is associated with earth. Refer to the trigrams of *heaven* and *Earth* shown in figure 12.3. (Note: The capitalization is being used to differentiate the primordial concept of Earth as related to heaven from the element earth in the five elements.)

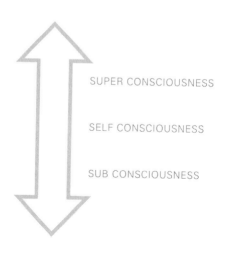

SUPER CONSCIOUSNESS

SELF CONSCIOUSNESS

SUB CONSCIOUSNESS

FIGURE 12.2   The Consciousness Gradient

Notice how the trigram for heaven is three solid yang lines, which reflect the ultimate pure state of yang (as an archetype of the original split of the Tao). Notice also how the Earth trigram has three yin lines, which represent the pure state of yin. These are the symbolic representations of the ultimate states of these two poles. Now, when we look at how they both interact in humans, we get the trigrams for fire and water (see figure 12.4).

The fire trigram resembles that of heaven except with a single yin line in the middle, which functions as the substance that fire needs to burn as fuel. The water trigram looks like the Earth trigram except for a single yang line in the middle, which gives water its power and dynamic life-carrying energy in our world. Bringing fire and water into balance with our intellect creates an environment for heaven and Earth to coexist in balance within our body. This becomes the fundamental basis of our alchemical work.

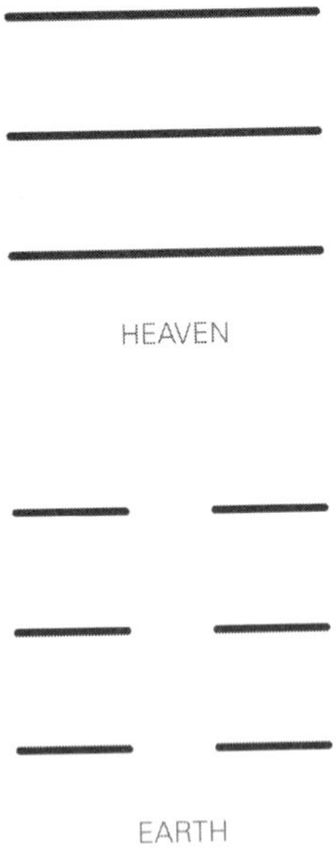

HEAVEN

FIRE

EARTH

WATER

FIGURE 12.3
The Pure Trigrams

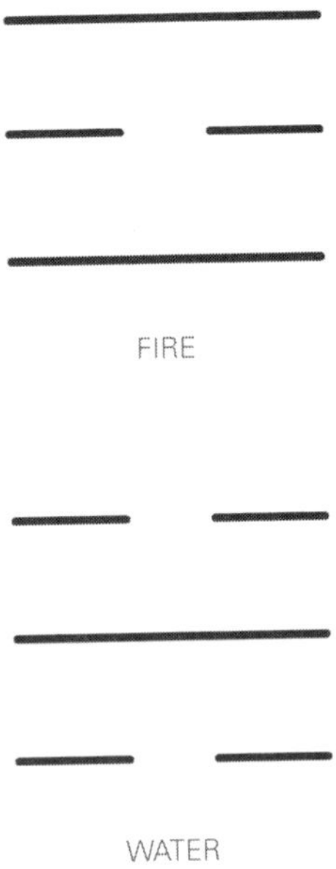

FIGURE 12.4
How Heaven and Earth Manifest
in Humans before Alchemy

We can take this information and overlay it to get to our next level of understanding of this system. The fusion of yin and yang takes place in the central earth element of the intellect, which acts as the pivot of the entire axis. They can come together if the space is clear in the center. Now, if we have not cleared an ample amount of the shadow "noise" in the intellect and/or if self-consciousness is afflicted by this, then we have a problem. Notice an interesting phenomenon—namely, that our self-consciousness and our superconsciousness *both* feed suggestions into our subconsciousness, as shown in figure 12.5. If we are constantly wrestling with aversions and cravings, we will keep channeling negative energy into the defense mechanisms we've created in our subconscious reasoning. These processes get programmed in and, in turn, feed belief systems and fear-inspired thoughts back into our self-conscious realm. This is the wrong way to go; it is this downward force-feeding that has gotten us into a real mess.

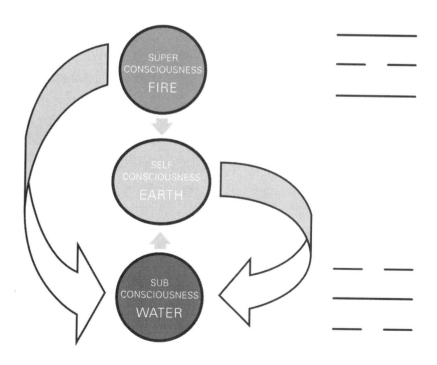

FIGURE 12.5   How Information Transfers in Human Consciousness

To better understand the differentiation of these levels, let's examine some of their characteristics (see table 12.1).

The most important concept to hold in mind here is that *the subconscious mind is amenable to suggestion.* These suggestions either form into shadow charges from our misunderstanding of life or come from conscious programming. In other words, our subconscious is taking programming either way; unless we are constantly engaged in what is passing through to it, someone, some insanity, or some demon will do it for us instead.

This is where our involvement comes in. It is absolutely imperative that we program what we want to see in our lives directly into our subconsciousness. At first, when we are primarily concerned with pulling weeds, these suggestions will come in the form of basic cognitive behavioral changes. This involves putting in healthy suggestions to override old bad habits that have been haunting us; it becomes a vital part of the process of deflating the energy of our shadow fields and pulling back our personal power.

For instance, say every time we see a car accident on the side of the road, we have a full panic attack because we remember the terrible accident that killed our parents when we were young. In this case, our internal healing work drives us to:

- Feel that energy once the thought field is invoked.

- Watch it with an open heart while pulling back all the power we've pumped into the fear of this event.

- Do our mental, emotional, and spiritual cleansing on the energy of this topic.

- Place a suggestion into our subconscious mind to be thankful for, in this example, having our parents as long as we did. We do this whenever we see an accident to automatically relax our system and secrete endorphins into our bloodstream.

TABLE 12.1   CONSCIOUSNESS ROAD MAP

ASPECT	SUPERCONSCIOUSNESS	SELF-CONSCIOUSNESS	SUBCONSCIOUSNESS
Element	Fire	Earth	Water
Manifesting Principle	Inspiration	Intellect	Intuition
Power	Attention / focus	Reasoning / integration	Intention/ willpower
Feeds Info to:	Sub- and self-consciousness	Subconsciousness	Self-consciousness
Gets Info from:	The Great Tao / Universal Intelligence	Super- and subconsciousness	Super- and self-consciousness

In essence, we place an "overlay" suggestion on top of the old one. We teach ourselves to be aware of these patterns, and then we place healthier habits into the subconscious mind as new programming to replace the old faulty "code." A word of caution, though: there is a yin and yang principle to everything (as we have learned), and this yang principle of actively reprogramming the mind has become quite fashionable in self-help circles lately. It is important to always maintain balance, and this means doing the reconciliation work. The yin aspect of this principle is the act of allowing us to *feel* and heal the traumas of the past. This leads to the deflation of the shadow energy. This work, by its very nature, is not particularly comfortable; if it were, then this content would never have been stuffed down into the shadow in the first place! A proper healing perspective requires *both* sides in order to accomplish the Great Work. We must heal our wounds and reclaim our power, while also implanting new behaviors and positive suggestions. Balance is the Way.

The subconscious mind will put into play anything we program into it once we become more adept at this game. We essentially create a blank canvas of our spiritual energy upon which to play. Working through the murky waters of our current subconscious shadow habits becomes quite fun when we finally get a grasp of this principle and start to literally "reprogram" our response patterns and habits. As we pull the weeds out of the dark corners of our energy fields, we get more and more self-conscious clarity, and we can use this to implant our subconsciousness with whatever goals, dreams, or aspirations we want. This is where the truly exciting part comes in.

With this knowledge, we can become active co-creators on the planet. We can picture the world and the life we want to see and help it take form and shape. The more we connect with our own internal power, the easier this process becomes and the quicker it continues to happen. I have met many people who are venerable wizards at this. They live the life of their dreams and enjoy all the world has to offer. The ones who stay happy are the ones who keep growing and evolving personally.

It has recently been popularized that people can learn this system and use it to crack the code of manifestation. They see themselves driving Bentleys to their boats and having several houses staffed with servants all around the planet. Whatever the material fantasy is, however, it is a small portion of the entirety of the human birthright. There is great danger in using this system only as a means to these ends. Sure, having material possessions is not inherently bad. In fact, go ahead and enjoy what the world has to offer, but—and here's the big but—to what end? What many of these systems have failed to impart is the most important aspect of this entire axis: the one that takes us from the realm of wizardry into that of enlightenment and sainthood.

The Law of Attraction

In the law of attraction, we are taught to focus on our desires and to realize that whatever we focus on becomes manifest. It teaches us to be careful where our attention goes because anything that we "plant" will grow. From a Taoist alchemical perspective, it essentially teaches us to take the desires of the wood element and tie our attention (fire) and intention (water) to it in order to make them manifest (see figure 12.6). It deals with the growth and aspiration side of human experience and attempts to make manifest the fulfillment of dreams and the empowerment of people through the proper understanding of universal laws. Human suffering, in this theory, comes from focusing our attention on what we do not want or on the lack of a certain thing we desire. Welcome to aversions and cravings! Essentially, this system is explaining parts of the same spiritual science we are learning here but in a very truncated form. Namely, it says that when we put energy into the lack or the opposite of a particular desire, we are feeding a cycle of suffering. Gaining clarity and understanding of this system will lead to "liberation."

This "liberation" leads to the liberation of our desires, and, yes, it certainly helps us understand how to pattern our life in a successful and healthy manner. However, it does not adequately address other elements of the human experience. First of all, the opposite pole of the horizontal axis is the metal element, which is responsible for the balancing and checking energy of decline and reduction. More of everything in perpetuity smells like the mark of Western cultural influence on spiritual science. Here, we have the story of the world being our oyster, which we have every right to ravish and enjoy fully. Sure we should enjoy things, of course, but *within reason*. Balance is the key, and tempering our desires and letting go of the past is counterpoint to a perpetual desire-driven mentality. Yes, human desires backed by strong emotion are a very powerful catalyst and an easy way to manifest things on the planet for ourselves. If we are not careful, however, they can lead us directly away from the main goal of our existence, which is self-realization and the evolution of our consciousness. The law of attraction, as taught, is an incredible tool for getting it partially right in the real world, but it is still a system based on imbalance. Always remember what the Great Tao wishes from its two offspring, yin and yang: balance and equality. In my opinion, the law of attraction needs to be tempered with a much grander motive—that of ultimate awakening. Seek true happiness.

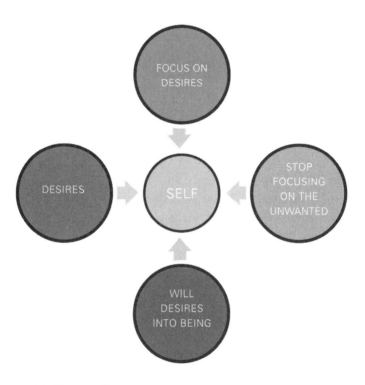

FIGURE 12.6   The Law of Attraction Using the Taoist Framework

The Superconscious Influence

The Western tradition speaks of the concept of revelation. This revelation is how God reveals himself to us in every instant. We are taught that it is our job to accept this reality gracefully and without judgment because it is perfect exactly how it is. This is a very good illustration of superconscious influence and our relationship to it. The Great Tao is all things and places and times, all at once. It is unfolding and spiraling in and out of existence in every instant. It accounts for all the cycles within cycles *within cycles* that account for the movement of the largest clusters of galaxies to the subatomic interactions going on in every cell of our bodies. The universe is so big that it is impossible to comprehend the scale—down from infinity and up to infinity. It seems that the farther (or deeper) we look, the more we keep finding more levels on even larger (and smaller) scales. It is absolutely beautiful and incredible, and it is awe-inspiring. We have recently ascertained that the universe seems to follow a specific type of mathematics that shows that everything follows a fractal pattern.[1] In essence, much like a hologram, even the smallest part has encoded in it the "blueprint" of the whole. We see this same phenomenon in the DNA of human beings. All the code from the start of life on this planet (and some would argue that it came from another planet) is encoded in every cell in our DNA. That means we have all the information *within* us that encodes our cells to become a fish, a tree, an ape, or a carrot. We have all the information in us right here and right now.

Jeremy Narby, an anthropologist who studied the spiritual ceremonies of Amazonian tribes, showed how the natives derive their profound understanding of herbal medicines. He explained that shamans mostly make the same claim about their profound understanding of herbalism—that is, the *plants told them*. In essence, Narby discovered that these natives, by ingesting a hallucinogenic brew called *ayahuasca* (DMT), communicate with the "coiled serpent," which *tells* them how to prepare the plants. He then postulated that we are all at a subconscious level of communication with *our own DNA* and that this communication is driving us to evolve and become more self-aware.[2] These shamans, by ingesting the brew, put themselves into a state where their self-conscious reasoning could observe the conversation that is always taking place between the superconscious realm and our subconscious realm (in this case, via our own DNA). The subconscious mind somehow understands this information and changes the way we express ourselves by switching certain genetic sequences on and off based on the messaging it receives.

It is also fascinating that we have recently discovered a whole internal system of language that involves the release of *photons* (particles of light) when our DNA zips and unzips.[3] The photons somehow communicate with the DNA in our cells, and a system of coordination instantly orchestrates our growth and direction based on this information. In other words, somehow, superconsciousness relays information to us via our DNA, and our subconsciousness then takes this information and encodes it into a photon-based language, which it instantly communicates to all the cells in our body. We also know that much of our genetic expression comes from the trillions of bacteria within us. It seems that life is having a profound conversation all around us. We instantly shift what it is we are doing, and we literally "create" a new reality based on this new encoding. This is where the magic happens.

Once we learn to *listen* to superconsciousness, we begin our resonant tuning with the primal will to the good of the entire universe. It seems that there is a definite *direction* in our evolution and that this has been encoded through our DNA, which has been driving us to become more self-aware since the very beginning.[4] However, that first moment when we became self-aware as humans also ushered us into polarity consciousness. Through the resultant reactions to our aversions and cravings that were born from this "fall," we began to create "noise" in the channel. We began feeding energy into the shadows of our subconscious reasoning, distorting the message or the light-based language that flows from super- to subconsciousness. We stopped hearing the inner voice and fell further and further into confusion. We became convinced that "this is it" and deluded ourselves that we had attained the highest level of evolution possible on the planet. This then forced us to invent tools and technologies to make up for the inherent powers we had forsaken. We thought we lost Eden, but all we really lost was our ability to see it. *We fell asleep and have been living a dream ever since.*

So, let's now look at the Taoist model for manifestation that corrects this deviant mentality and puts us back on the fast track to evolution and freedom. Walking with the Tao is like a hot knife through butter. It is like *effortlessly* flowing down the stream of all that is because we are in sync with the superconscious fractal of which we are a central part. This model for manifestation is the correction for our human pathology; when properly understood and practiced, it will result in nothing short of illumination and true self-realization.

The development of our correct understanding of the nature of our existence leads us to dissolve the egos of our self-conscious identities and literally "step aside" and allow superconsciousness to feed information directly into our subconsciousness. This, in turn, makes our self-consciousness the willing agent of the universal mind. Notice in figure 12.7 how the information of the subconscious mind channels directly into the self-conscious mind and vice versa. The master along the path is selfless and takes inspiration from the living currents

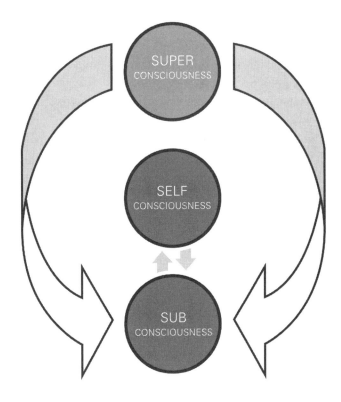

FIGURE 12.7   Letting the Tao Guide Our Actions

of the Tao and acts in harmony with these currents. He is, however, capable of communicating and interacting with the superconsciousness *through* his subconscious mind. He can still implant seeds for growth and manifest his intentions in reality because of his access to and understanding of the internal language. His renewed understanding of the relationship of the self-conscious and subconscious minds creates a "rebirth" of sorts as he shakes off the heavy influences of the shadow and wakes up to his true potential and place in the universe. Life then becomes a dynamic act of "playing" like a child out in nature—full of wonderment and magic.

PERSONAL JOURNEYS Fireflies in Machu Picchu

I had spent a number of days hiking the *Camino Inca*, which was the original trail from the city of Cusco into Machu Picchu, Peru. It was quite the adventure, and the ruins of Machu Picchu were absolutely incredible. I had spent an entire day wandering around, as it is an enormous site with plenty to see. After having made friends with a local guide, I was told that the park would reopen later that night for visitors. I found some food and had to wait around for several hours before I could go back in. There were only two sets of couples and myself waiting when the gates opened that night. We paid our money, and I let the others work their way into the park with their flashlights first. I wanted to go in the dark and *see* with my shen.

Once I was all alone, there was an eerie silence. Machu Picchu is a big place, and here I was, standing alone in the dark with an uncomfortable feeling rising up. I then asked God to guide me: "You brought me here, now tell me what to do!" I couldn't believe my eyes. A firefly lit up right in front of me and then started floating along the path. I followed dutifully until the light flickered out. There I was standing in complete darkness again. Now what? Another firefly (it could have been the same one) lit up and continued to travel away from me. Again I followed.

I must have followed a chain of a few dozen of these until they stopped lighting up. I looked around and found myself in the center of the central temple on the main hill! There was an incredible glow to the night sky, almost as if it was flashing. I could hear and actually *feel* voices and a dull chant permeating the air. The other visitors were nowhere to be seen. I sat with my back against one wall of the temple and began to meditate.

I was young at the time, twenty-three years old. I remember feeling overwhelmed by the whole experience. I kept telling myself to trust in Higher Power. I could sense a stream of information dumping into my head. Every time I tried to focus on it, it felt like I was being bounced out of there. A voice in my head that I distinctly recognized simply told me not to worry about it, that this information was to unlock and open up for me at some point in the future. I was too young to grasp it all then.

I relaxed and allowed whatever was happening to happen. I felt pings and pangs throughout my body and just settled in to be passive about the whole thing. Obviously, my superconsciousness was in a serious dialogue with my subconsciousness, and I was not allowed to hear the details. It was as if my self-conscious mind did not have the expanded sense of Self or the capacity to deal with the information that was being transmitted. There was too much of "me," or who I thought I was, in the way. I sat silently and allowed, part in curiosity and part in utter terror.

To this day, I don't quite know what happened when I woke up. I felt a jolt and found myself lying on my back as if I had just fallen backward. I got up and was perplexed about where I was. It took me a couple of minutes of exploring to realize that I was on the *other side* of the wall I had been sitting against. Did I actually fall through that wall? Did I get up and wander around but not remember it? Either way, I felt strongly that it was time to go. My work there was done, or perhaps Machu Picchu was done with me. I was told that I'd be back a few years later, but it was now time for me to move on. Right then, there was a flash of a firefly in front of me.

I dutifully followed the chain of lights and eventually found myself back outside by the gate. They had guided me into the ruins and then had guided me out. The night guard gave me a smirk and asked if I had enjoyed myself. I tried to crack a smile but simply kept walking; I had a lot to think about.

It is important to remember that this level of mastery is born out of our understanding that comes from our reconciliation of the primordial split of yin and yang. We are still talking of uniting poles along a spectrum with super- and subconsciousness coming together in a synergistic relationship. This is the essence of the Tao of manifestation, and it is the mark of liberation. The system does not stop here, however. The Great Work of Taoist alchemy specifically takes this level of understanding to its natural conclusion. We are to literally *become* the understanding of this phenomenon. Having a mental understanding of a concept in a theoretical form is wonderful, but it will eventually lead to disharmony as it is a still a polarization of the Tao. We must learn to fully *embody* this understanding and *become* this understanding in a very real sense, so that we may then fully bring balance to our realization and not depart off into levels of abstraction.

The Fusion of Fire and Water

The vertical axis that links attention and intellect (figure 6.1) is a symbolic depiction of how the levels of consciousness interact. Consequently, we can come to understand how to use this system for our own liberation. The split of consciousness is wonderful for our third-dimensional brain to understand, but it is also important to note that the central premise of the Great Work is the *union* of fire and water—the *dissolution* of the perception of duality. The Tao is One. In our path of return to the Source, we must reconcile all understanding of the alchemical science and, in the end, dissolve all levels of duality and literally *become* what we are practicing.

With the artificial construct of the "self" (which is the ego) dissolved, the fusion of fire and water becomes the literal fusion of super- and subconsciousness (see figure 12.8). This means there is no separation between us and the Great Tao. There is no interference or noise that disrupts this flow, and we are fully connected all the time. We become the very embodiment of the life force that moves through all things, and yet "we" as we know ourselves no longer exist. What we used to identify ourselves as—our defense mechanisms, our fear-inspired behavior, our material desires—washes away as the light of awareness is turned inward. As we illuminate the dark corners of our shadows, we remove all the skeletons from our closets and "come clean," seeing reality for what it is in the current moment. At this point, we become the agents for the universal will, which flows *through* us as we are constantly connected to it from *within*. Actually, at this stage, *we are it*. Our realization of what and how special we truly are is no longer jaded by self-doubt or self-aggrandizement. We finally realize what reality truly is and where we belong within it. We are no longer the embodiment of the primordial separation; rather, we are the embodiment of the *union* that is the end of the Great Work. We don't lose our identity; instead, we actually *find* our true identity. Our unique identity is an important part of how the Tao manifests, so don't worry about that part—all the good stuff that makes you special remains!

This Great Work is the subject of the next chapter, which is about the Light Body. This Light Body is the "homecoming" or the full-circle understanding of the alchemical process. Our embodiment of this new

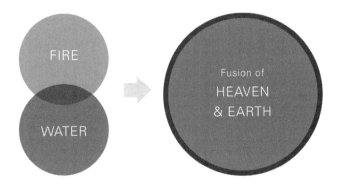

FIGURE 12.8   The Alchemical Path

comprehension becomes the final aim because of one important fact: the ultimate step is to *become* the realization of which we speak. The Great Work is the process through which we apply the realization of the principles in this chapter to our physical body. Remember, our body is only "separate" from our mind, emotions, and spirit because of polarity consciousness. The wax of the candle and the aura of the flame are simply opposite poles of the *same realization*, and one needs the other to complete the cycle. The fusion of the five elements and the reformation of yin and yang is the process by which we literally work and clean inside our own body until we are fully linked up and healed. The more we connect our subconscious and superconscious minds by learning to listen internally and to clear away the noise, the more we *become* that very realization.

We are now ready to study the "graduate level" subject matter. This is the fulfillment of the Great Work and the embodiment of the union of yin and yang.

13

THE BIRTH OF THE LIGHT BODY

The light is neither inside not outside the self. . . .
Once you turn the light around, everything in the world is turned around.

LÜ TUNG PIN, *The Secret of the Golden Flower* (translated by Thomas Cleary)

Famed Inca shaman and scholar Alberto Villoldo coined the term *Homo luminous* to describe the next level of humanity's advancement on this planet. We are in the very process of the evolution of our species from *Homo sapiens* to *Homo luminous*.[1] Although this coming progression is the ancient, stated birthright of all humans as taught by a number of worldly traditions, it has, until recently, been a lost spiritual technology for many centuries. This knowledge has fortunately re-emerged for the masses. *Homo luminous* is the result of the practice of all yoga (which means "union") and is the natural consequence to our illumination. The more aware we become, the clearer the Light Body practice continues to be for us. The more we wake up, the more we can see the energy fields and luminous bodies of others and eventually ignite our eternal Light Bodies.

We are becoming increasingly aware of the energetic makeup of our universe, while our science is coming full circle in proving that consciousness is the central aspect of *everything*. In fact, just as space and time are tied into the rhythms of all movement, the expansion and collapse of our universe from the big bang theory looks remarkably like the Hindu story of Lord Brahma breathing in and out—contracting and expanding the whole universe in this cycle. So, if there is no real concept of time except in how it relates to the space it is associated with within the fractal, then what's fifteen billion years among friends? In other words, it's all a big dream. These vast expanses of time and space that we calculate outward (toward the edge of the universe) and inward (looking into the subatomic world) are simply scales that blow our rational and ordered three-dimensional minds away. However, they also mean absolutely nothing to our consciousness, which is in all places at all times.

As we start to wake up to the many mysteries of our universe that exist outside *and* inside our bodies, we learn that each of us has a critical and central role to play in the grand scheme of this shared existence. We are intimately connected to all that is, and we are the willful agents of the natural patterns of the One life force. Yet, we feel trapped—trapped within these physical bodies and further trapped in the dramas of our shadow energies. We feel drained and disconnected and always wonder why we are so lost. *Until now.*

Now we have studied the essence of the Taoist alchemical teaching and have come to understand the nature of suffering. More important, we have learned to clean up our energy fields and free our minds from the turmoil of our shadow energies. We have also learned to unlock our blocked energy flow and to return the powers of our subconscious mind back to their intimate connection with superconsciousness. We, in short, have gleaned the knowledge to identify our problems, correct the disharmonies that exist within us, and tune into the pure energies of nature that are available to us, while also reprogramming healthy habits into our energy fields. We should finally be complete, right?

Not exactly. For within this newfound ability to awaken ourselves, there exists a paradoxical void. Soon after we have learned the tools to break from our trance state and plot our own course, we are being told to surrender to the superconscious will and become a participating agent of this consciousness. We then discover that we must do this work and dissolve our egos so that the intelligence of the Tao can guide us freely through the world as conscious co-creators of reality. This sounds very good and passive, but you are probably wondering, *What do I do now?*

We have now arrived at the fundamental paradox of the Taoist teachings. We learned early on that it is our "doing" that creates most of our problems, and we have learned to practice "nondoing" or "being" in our mental meditations. This practice is very helpful in showing us the following:

- The insanity under which we operate under daily

- How we needn't engage in it

- How liberating it is to passively "be" without reacting to myriad events and circumstances all the time

This is where the first breakthrough in our "doing pathology" comes in. When we practice nonaction and really find that space and are comfortable there, eventually, well . . . we get hungry. Or we have to go to the bathroom. Maybe our legs start to hurt from sitting, and we need to walk around and stretch. We get up to do so, and we see a hummingbird outside, so we watch it and smile. While in the garden, a neighbor says hello and invites us to come watch a video recommended by a friend, and we do so. The clip is about polar bears dying in the Arctic, and we are moved. The following week a cousin asks us to get involved in a group that helps raise awareness about global warming, and we attend. There we meet the love of our life and get married. Now, together, we travel to exotic places and try to make a difference . . . following reality's lead the whole way through. Again, the Western concept of revelation comes through here. The Great Tao has placed our path in front of us right here and right now. We are so mentally abstract about the meaning of life and what we're supposed to do that we don't see the path right in front of us. We wear out our brake pads and drain our vitality instead of enjoying the ride.

So, the first aspect of "nondoing" is to free the mind and energy from the grips of the shadow and really enjoy the present moment for what it truly is. All the grace and beauty in the world presents itself to us when we do. This does not, however, account for the paradoxical effort required to complete the Great Work. So, how do we reconcile the laissez-faire Taoist approach of noneffort with the dedicated work ethic of "the Way is the Training"?

My grand master studied diligently in a monastery in China for several years, starting in his childhood. There was a great deal of physical labor and chores, along with several hours a day of horse stance. This deep kung fu stance helps drop the energy down to the lower dantien while strengthening the legs and building resolve—zhi in the kidneys. This is part of the very tedious training that is done for at least one year before the young monks are even allowed to learn to throw their first punch. The tradition of kung fu literally translates to "hard work" or "eat bitter" in Chinese. So, how were these high-level Taoist adepts conducting such rigorous physical training with incredible dedication and still learning to relax? How did they deal with the two axioms of "Taoist Way Not Forced" and "The Way Is the Training" in the same curriculum? Again, we see the central paradox of Taoist training and one that needs to be teased out before we go any further.

There is an inherent level of distortion that we humans begin with when we incarnate here on Earth. Assuming we have perfectly adjusted families and very little drama growing up, we still have the essential human mental pathology to deal with—the nature of suffering and our leaking of energy to our shadows through aversions and cravings. This is why monasteries like to take children in before a certain age—there is less junk to deal with. So, let's assume that most of us didn't grow up in a temple setting deep in the Himalayas and that we, instead, grew up in the West, with all the insanity that comes with such an upbringing. At this point, we have a good amount of emotional charge and mental aversions that have fed our power into our shadows. We have done our damage and have a good deal of work to complete in order to "undo" that which has been done.

Recall from the chapter about the nature of suffering that we discussed the notion of karma and how it equates simply to "action." You will probably concede that a good amount of "action" has gone into our shadow processes over the years. In fact, we've come a long way to create an enormous mess (unconsciously). Although we can practice "nonaction" for several years to dissipate the charge we have stored there, the ancient Taoist masters have found that a fusion works better for the majority of the people they encounter—especially in the West. Sure, an occasional student has a sudden flash of insight and, through this enlightenment, instantly clears herself of all the junk she was carrying and is free. But this is very rare, and too few people experience this. What about the rest of us? Well, we get to work. The same aspect of karma comes in as we instill *positive* karma into our lives. We develop rituals and habits that help *remind* us every day—actually several times a day—to do one simple thing: WAKE UP! We keep falling asleep to the deep trances burned into our shadows, and so we must set constant reminders and perform practices that illuminate our awareness of this phenomenon. This is an incredibly powerful and effective way for us to attain real results in a short amount of time.

In this realization, the paradox is resolved. We work hard in the training in order to erase *previous* "work" that we have done and to function as a failsafe against falling back asleep. We *simultaneously* practice "nonaction" as related to our mental and emotional attachments, while we develop our strong energy fields. We also clear the power trapped in our shadows, while we learn to observe reality for what it truly is. We comprehend what it means to *relax* in our effort—we fuse *action* and *inaction*, just as we balance yin and yang. We train to relax in a deep horse stance, and we study to stay relaxed until the moment of a necessary strike . . . or until we actually have to stand in front of those people at that presentation. We understand how to be aware of our energy flow and stop the leaking. Doing so, we gather more personal power and cultivate further awareness of the living, breathing currents of the Tao flowing through us. We essentially wake up to a deep understanding of who we truly are and continue cultivating and refining our energy toward the ultimate aim, which is the development of the Light Body and its eventual ignition.

The Light Body in Different Traditions

In this section, we will conduct a brief overview of the various cultures on the planet that have a Light Body tradition. This is in no way a complete list; rather, it serves as a sampling of the range and thoroughness of this body of knowledge across the globe. The take-home message is that dozens of cultures have been involved in this type of training for thousands of years. This is a very serious field of study with a rich history. It has slipped under the cultural radar in the modern age for reasons discussed earlier but is now in resurgence. The more we wake up, the more we become interested in this spiritual science again. We are slowly remembering what we thought had been lost.

I have chosen small excerpts from each and have kept it brief, as this book is not intended to be a cross-cultural analysis of the intricacies of the varying practices. Consider the following a primer covering differing views of the same subject; see it as an open invitation for you to delve deeper into whichever tradition appeals to you the most.

EGYPT

The Egyptian tradition of the Light Body is one we wish we had more information about. Although a number of living cultures around the world have preserved the Light Body tradition, the traditions of the Egyptian and Mayan cultures of antiquity have all but disappeared and are now being reconstructed by historians and anthropologists. We do, however, have a powerful vision left behind by the priesthood of this ancient tradition, and it is that of the ascending Light Body and the nature of "star fields" located in interstellar space.

Here is an excerpt from a manual on Egyptian magic:

> The Egyptians divided man's constitution into a graduated series of parts. First was the physical body, or *khat*. Overshadowing, or enveloping, this body was a series of subtle bodies, each more ethereal than the last. The first of these, and the most dense of the subtle bodies, was the shadow, or *khaibit*. The next was the *ka*, the body of emotions. This was followed by the heart, *ab* (or *hati-ab*, which can be translated "outer heart"). The next was the *ba* (soul), which was linked to the *ka* through the *ab*. The *ba* rested in the spirit-body, or *sah* (sometimes *sahu*), which was presided over by the spirit, or *khu*. . . . These and other designations for man's components were all governed by the highest, the *khabs*, the divine component which means star. . . .

The magician's Subtle Body, or Body of Light, is the chief
tool used in some Low Magick operations and in almost
all High Magick operations. Essentially, it is the living aura
that pervades the physical body and extends slightly beyond
it. It is shaped somewhat like an oval or egg, . . . and it
contains colorful swirling forces of energy that express
thoughts and emotions.[2]

We can obviously see some similarities in this conceptual framework with
that of the Taoist system we have been discussing. The Egyptians were
known to have a very cohesive system, with a strong underground order
that preserved this information for centuries. Much of this Egyptian
knowledge has been preserved through a number of present-day orders
in the West.

TIBET

The Tibetans have one of the best-documented and clear-cut histories
of the Light Body practice. There are a number of practitioners alive
to this day who are intimately involved in this work and who serve
as living bearers of this tradition. Although a great deal of chaos and
destruction has been inflicted on the country of Tibet, much of the
tradition has been preserved outside the country, and for this, we are
eternally grateful.

The following is an excerpt from Norbu Rinpoche:

The *Jalu* (in Tibetan), or Body of Light, realized through
the practice of Dzogchen is different from the *Gyulu*, or
Illusory Body, realized through the practices of the Higher
Tantras. The Gyulu is dependent on the subtle prana of
the individual, and thus, since prana is always considered
to be of the relative dimension in Dzogchen, this Gyulu is
not considered to be Total Realization. The Jalu, or Body
of Light, itself, is a way of manifesting realization that is
particular to the masters who have carried the practice of
the Longde or of the Mennagde to their ultimate level, and

with only very short breaks in the lineage, it has continued to be manifested right up to the present day.[3]

Master Norbu then proceeded to tell a tale of a certain master who had decided that it was time to die. The master asked his disciples to seal him in a tent and leave him in peace for seven days:

> The disciples went down the mountain, and waited, camped at the foot of it for seven days, during which time it rained a great deal, and there were many rainbows. Then they went back up and opened the tent, which was sewn up just as they had left it. All that they found inside was the master's clothes, his hair, and his fingernails and toenails. His clothes were the clothes of a lay person, and they remained there in a heap where he had been sitting, with the belt still wrapped around the middle. He had left them just like a snake sheds a skin.[4]

The Tibetans have a long history of cultivation of what they call the Rainbow Body. They have dedicated practices devoted to this, with thousands of aspirants who train in these systems. Their great masters were said to have been able to consciously shed the remnants of their physical bodies and to evolve into a body of pure light.

CHINA

The Taoists of China have one of the longest-standing traditions of alchemy and Light Body work in the world. Like Tibet, much of this work has been diligently documented in the Taoist Canon, and a great deal of this information still lives in the oral tradition. Masters impart this wisdom on their students only when they are ready and can finally undergo the final illumination processes.

An extraordinary level of detail has been transferred along these lines within the Chinese tradition, where there certainly is no shortage of words. Here is an example of an excerpt in the preparation of the "immortal fetus":

Gather the five vitalities and return them to the source (the
upper tan t'ien in the brain) where the union of (positive
and negative) vitalities will produce the immortal foetus.
. . . If the five vitalities are full, a golden light will soar up
to unite with the light of (essential) nature to become a
single light which is the union of the radiant vitality of the
positive principle (yang) in the head and the bright light of
the negative principle (yin) in the abdomen into one single
light which will result in the egress from the immortal
foetus. The practiser should then lower his eyes slowly to
look down before closing them with the combined force of
his heart and intellect as if to make a jump.[5]

There are volumes and volumes of very specific instruction on how
to go through this process and what pitfalls to avoid. Needless to say,
this is the primary tradition from which I teach, and this excerpt is
not to be taken out of context. It serves merely as an illustration of
the depth of scholarship that has gone into this very specific field by
thousands of practitioners.

It is important to remember that there is *one Light Body* and that
the various traditions of the world have come to describe it in slightly
different ways. I personally found the Taoist path to be very well laid
out and easy to follow as a student. This, in no way, should take away
from the validity of the other systems that exist. In fact, I have studied many of them, and each holds a special piece of the puzzle in my
opinion. With a history of secrecy and distortion in some of these
traditions, bits and pieces of this vast body of knowledge are often
missing. In fact, there is a great deal of this in the Chinese culture,
as everybody tries to preserve their own turf of this "ancient Chinese
secret." In the old days, this knowledge was supreme power for a clan
or tribe, and the secrets were carefully guarded.

My grand master, who is a traditionally trained Chinese man without a hippie bone in his body, had an interesting response to a student
when asked who the originator of our knowledge was. His answer:
"Atlantis." All the jaws dropped in the room; with further thought,
however, it made sense. Each of these spheres of understanding that

sprang up around the world, when looked at as a whole, points to a previous era when we allegedly had a cohesive body of knowledge that revolved around these practices before we fell into darker times. We are now waking up to this knowledge again.

INDIA

The Hindu tradition is also noted for its exceptional scholarship in this field and its priceless contribution to the yogic arts. Hindu scholars represent an unbroken line of Vedic scholarship and research and are another of the "flame holder" traditions of the world. They have an extensive understanding of the energy systems that operate in the body, and their knowledge of yoga and breathwork speaks for itself.

Here is a piece from Paramahansa Yogananda's autobiography:

> So long as the soul of man is encased in one, two, or three body-containers, sealed tightly with the corks of ignorance and desires, he cannot merge with the Sea of Spirit. When the gross physical receptacle is destroyed by the hammer of death, the other two coverings—astral and causal—still remain to prevent the soul from consciously joining the Omnipresent Life. When desirelessness is attained through wisdom, its power disintegrates the two remaining vessels. The tiny human soul emerges, free at last; it is one with the Measureless Amplitude. . . . When a soul is out of the cocoon of the three bodies it escapes forever from the law of relativity and becomes the ineffable Ever-Existent. Behold the butterfly of Omnipresence, its wings etched with stars and moons and suns![6]

When we first start to study these systems, one thing becomes quite apparent from the start: *there's a lot going on here!* There are people (very intelligent ones, I may add) who devote their entire lives to the study of these systems. There are precious few, however, who combine such rigorous intellectual study with the actual *practice* of these arts. That being said, a great number of the most famous ascended masters who have walked the Earth in this past cycle have come from India. India, to this day, remains the world's treasure chest of spiritual knowledge and the holy men and women who practice it. This is a country where God permeates all daily activities and colors all traditions.

INCA

There is very little left of the living Inca tradition, thanks to the Spanish conquest. This once-great empire was known for its stargazers and medicine men, along with the incredible architecture of its monuments. A small number of shamans have come down from the high Andes recently, however, and have begun teaching the knowledge of the ancient Inca. They feel that with the coming Earth changes, it is time for us to come together and relearn what we once knew about the luminous body. Dr. Alberto Villoldo has played an integral part in bringing this knowledge to the West. Here is an excerpt from one of his books on the subject:

> The luminous energy field is shaped like a doughnut
> (known in geometry as a torus) with a narrow axis or
> tunnel, less than a molecule thick, in the center. In the
> Inka language, it is known as the *popo*, or luminous bubble.
> Persons who have had near-death experiences report
> traveling through this tunnel in their return voyage to the
> light. The human energy field is a mirror of the Earth's
> magnetic field, which streams out of the North Pole and
> circumnavigates the planet to reenter again through the
> South Pole. Similarly, the flux lines or *cekes* of the luminous
> energy field travel out the top of the head and stream
> around the luminous body, forming a great oval the width
> of our outstretched arms. Our energy fields penetrate the
> Earth about twelve inches, then reenter the body through
> the feet.[7]

It is amazing how similar this is all starting to sound! The Inca tradition is having an incredible resurgence with the teaching of this knowledge.

JUDAIC-CHRISTIAN-ISLAMIC TRADITIONS

The origins of the religions of the "Book of Abraham" come from the ancient Zoroastrian and Egyptian traditions and their contemporaries. The early Judaic mystical knowledge fell under the umbrella of the study of the Kabala, which was essentially borrowed from earlier Egyptian knowledge. Much of the essence of this tradition carried over into Christianity and Islam, which have both maintained their own secret societies. The use of the halo as a device to convey association with divinity is described in the following quote:

> The whole-body image of radiance is sometimes called the "aureole" or *glory*; it is shown radiating from all round the body, most often of Christ or Mary, occasionally of saints (especially those reported to have been seen surrounded by one). Such an aureola is often a mandorla ("almond-shaped" vesica piscis), especially around Christ in Majesty, who may well have a halo as well. In depictions of the Transfiguration a more complicated shape is often seen, especially in the Eastern Orthodox tradition, as in the famous fifteenth-century icon in the Tretyakov Gallery in Moscow.[8]

The artistic depictions always show enlightened saints in their Light Bodies, emanating Divine Light through their mere presence. The story of the transfiguration of Enoch serves as a great example of this: "In the Book of Enoch, when Enoch returns to Earth, he tells his children that although they see him as the earthly, human Enoch, there is likewise an angelic Enoch (Metatron) that has stood in the Lord's Presence."[9] Enoch's developed Light Body allowed him to present in human form to his counterparts while being able to stand in the "Lord's presence." In this story, Enoch had been able to cross the bounds of three-dimensional reality with his understanding and development of a Luminous Body.

A great deal of Christian iconography portrays Jesus in the central role of the sun among our zodiac. In fact, there are thousands of references to Jesus being the *living embodiment* of the Guiding Light. There is a growing research that points to the parallels between Jesus, the Son of God, and our central star, the Sun of God.[10] It seems that much has been borrowed from the older Egyptian idea of sun worship and the notion of star seeding. If Jesus is to serve as an example for us in life, then the cultivation and *ignition* of the Light Body becomes the central goal of our religious practice. The understanding of our essential nature leads to the "en*light*enment" of our energy fields and the activation of our Light Body.

Coming Home

If Jesus Christ was to be understood as the "sun" versus the "son" of God, then what does that story mean to us? If the Egyptian mystery traditions speak of the Earth as being a literal "star seed," then where do we go from here? The emergence of an enlightened human is a spectacular thing. It bends time and space and creates something special. If Earth were a school and we were students, well, there are too few graduates right now. What does graduation from the Earth school mean? How can we understand what all these traditions are saying, and how can we relate to this information?

The answer is simple. *We already know.*

If we look at the concepts and principles we have studied thus far in this book, we can come to realize that we deal with a certain energy "exchange" every day of our lives. We have learned to maximize the flow of that energy through our field and to minimize the impedance, or the blocked flow, of that energy. We have learned to reclaim the power we, and only we, have trapped in our shadows, and we have come to understand the process by which our demons are created and shared with one another. Now, the reversal of this process leads us to an interesting place. Jesus teaches his disciples to "be a light unto thyselves," and we see similar language in several biblical passages:

> "Let your light so shine before men, that they may see your good works, and glorify your Father which is in heaven." —Matthew 5:16

> "While ye have light, believe in the light, that ye may be the children of light." —John 12:36

"For ye were sometimes darkness, but now are ye light in the Lord: walk as children of light." —Ephesians 5:8

We also hear the same theme from the Buddha:

"Be a light unto yourself, betake yourselves to no external refuge. Hold fast to the Truth. Look not for refuge to anyone but yourselves." —The Buddha, upon his deathbed

This is exactly what we are heading toward. By turning the light of awareness inward, we are able to experience the wonderment and mysteries of the universe through our alchemical process. We are able to free up more and more energy and to *refine* it into a better understanding of reality as it is. This refinement process frees up the smooth flow of energy in our outer meridians and opens up our eight extraordinary meridians, which lead to greater psychic intuition and inner vision. This level of attainment prepares us for the next step of our process, which is the fusion of yin and yang at every level of our energy system.

We begin by developing and balancing the lower dantien. Once consolidated and strong, we then use this energy to open, refine, and balance the energy of the middle dantien, whose place is around the heart. Again, after more practice, we do the same at the upper dantien (third eye) and then the crown. From here, there is very specific breathwork that allows us to create what is called, in Taoist lore, "the Immortal Fetus." This is an energy field that we cultivate and nurture daily. With rigorous effort and focused attention, we energetically birth this new body from within. Once this new body is created, we effectively molt off our physical attachment with the third dimension and allow for this new vehicle to become the transdimensional house for our expanded consciousness. At this point, many masters have been able to perform miraculous feats because they are no longer bound by the "laws" of the third dimension. Babaji and Lü Tung Pin, among many other ascended masters, have the ability to incarnate as they wish and take on any physical form that suits them. These ascended masters have no filter or distortion between what they wish and what is instantly manifest. They have literally evolved into *our birthright*—they have become examples of *Homo luminous*.

Now, the actual practice that is involved in creating the Light Body is beyond the scope of this book, as it is very detailed and requires years of practice and cultivation before attempting. In essence, all the groundwork laid out in this book must be mastered, and the student should have a great deal of proficiency in qi gong and internal awareness. Once the light of awareness is turned inward and the mysteries are unlocked, the path to the Light Body presents itself, and the student will be guided there. In fact, there is never a time when we are not being guided internally by our superconscious mind via our DNA. It seems that evolution has a trajectory, and we are the canvas. The Light Body is the *next* level in our growth. It is important to remember that it keeps on going from there. Once we become self-aware and develop a vehicle that *immortalizes our consciousness*, we keep growing and becoming more self-aware from there. Remember, in an ever-moving fractal, there really is no end—finite thinking is a mark of our polarity consciousness. It just gets more and more interesting; unfortunately, most humans don't even know the game!

I'd like to take a quick moment to comment on the statement "immortalizes our consciousness," because I feel it is an important one. It is said in the Hindu tradition that when we incarnate here on Earth, we agree to have our perfect memories "wiped" so that we can experience finding ourselves all over again. With each successive reincarnation, we take on new lessons and work toward a self-awareness cumulatively until we are finally "there." We break through and realize our true nature and are enlightened. With the evolution of *Homo luminous*, however, we essentially break the cycle of birth and death, as we no longer need our physical bodies to "exist" on this third-dimensional Earth anymore. We, in essence, will have come full circle and will have married yin and yang to *become* an active constituent of the Great Tao. It is said that an ascended human is a sight for sore eyes in other dimensional realms. This may have something to do with the low number of graduates we've had in the past five thousand years, or maybe it is because this is the central proving ground for everything. We are it, though. This is our time, and we have a small window within which to wake up and evolve or perish and take the ecosystem down with us.

I was subjected to a number of intense experiences as a monk. Many of these involved delving deeply into my inner realms and freeing trapped energy from my past. After one particular episode of heavy "rebirthing" type breathing with my teacher, I had pulled through a very difficult memory from my childhood. I had felt as if I were dying, and I wanted *anything* other than what I was feeling come up. Talk about aversions and cravings! After some initial struggle, I relaxed through it and simply let the feelings, memories, and thoughts be as they were and pass. Instead of dying, I felt liberated on the other side of this experience. It was as if I had shed forty spiritual pounds in that moment. I then lay there for some time before opening my eyes and trying to orient myself to the room. What I saw made me jump backward. Not only could I see a fully developed luminous egg around my teacher, but I could also see orbs of light around the other students on the far side of the room. As I started to squint my eyes and look at the details of their light bodies, I noticed another one that was brighter than and somewhat different from the others. As I tried to recognize his face, I realized that it wasn't one of my fellow monks. He had the glowing face of an old Chinese master. My teacher whispered to me that he was here to oversee our work and was a "friend" from the lineage. The master smiled at me and then walked right through the wall. I turned to my fellow students in awe and noticed that I could still see their light bodies. I thought that it was a hallucination. Little did I know that this was just the beginning of an adventure that I am still happily on.

The Light Body practice starts with the concepts and principles laid out in this book. But unless we start by building our foundations and working from the core upward, we will not be able to do it. It simply will not work. We cannot ignore any aspect of ourselves and expect to move on to the shiny, fuzzy stuff. We cannot avert the pain we sense lurking in our shadows and "leap" ahead for a Light Body without crashing down. This is classical trance consciousness. Don't fall for any shiny shortcuts! Once we can clearly see within and have a stable and strong foundation, we can then move to complete the Great Work. To evolve into *Homo luminous*, we need to bring super- and subconsciousness together through a healthy intellect that is free from attachments. We need to let the directionality of the life force guide us internally in order to grow and evolve and literally transform into the next iteration of our species.

I'd like to take a moment now to speak to a point that all critical minds come across when they read this type of material (I did as well): if there are guys and gals out there with Light Bodies, then why don't they come onto TV and show themselves? In the East, there are constant visitations and stories of people being accosted by masters. Even in the West, many are approached in the dream state and given instruction—but seldom in person and hardly ever in the public arena. However, through personal communication with the great "immortals" of my lineage, I have come to understand that there is a profound psychological flaw in the West that keeps these Light Bodies from appearing in this age—namely, that of the savior complex.

In short, the great ascended masters will not show up on prime-time TV and do that dance for you because, chances are, we'll expect them to fix all our problems, and then we'll put them up on a cross. However, it is quite common for them to appear to communicate with those of us who begin doing the work and who learn to "listen." The trap is this though: *they* do not matter in this process. They can show us the way until we find our own way, but they have already left us these wonderful systems to follow. Once we start to wake up, they and the entire rest of the universe are right here and right now.

The role of the masters is to illuminate the Way for those around them by the mere nature of a simple principle—their actual presence illuminates the darkness of ignorance. It is for us to become the light and literally "ignite" our Light Bodies into being. From here, our singular presence helps dispel the shadows around us and shine away ignorance. The breeding ground of vampires and zombies goes away when the light shines all around. The more people wake up, the easier the task of illumination gets, and the more pleasant our world becomes. We are in need of several "beacons" of light who will lead their lives by example and serve as inspiration for the family and friends around them. Shine into your world and make it a better place. The only way to do that is to change *yourself*. When we become *Homo luminous*, we set an example for the world around us; we needn't preach, and we needn't argue with people about doctrines or philosophy. Our mere presence will serve as an example of what liberated humanity looks like.

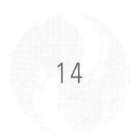

14

WHERE WE GO FROM HERE

We must be the change we wish to see in the world.

Often attributed to MAHATMA GANDHI

Coming full circle is the Taoist way, because everything is already here and now. So, the question then becomes, Why do we start the journey to begin with? Why do we do anything or go anywhere if there's really nothing to do or nowhere to go? The answer is simple. As yin and yang represent the primal split of Tao, this perceived split created all movement in the universe. With polarity comes spin, and with spin comes the movement and the breath of life in its myriad forms and faces. Coming home is our opportunity to finally let go of our own created dramas and fortified shadow energy and to move with the flow of the Tao. This is where we encounter the paradox of inaction versus action. It's like saying surfers do nothing once they catch a wave or that a sailboat does nothing when it is lined up behind a strong tail wind. The universe moves. The Great Tao moves. Being silent and still gives us a chance to harmonize with this movement and to literally "ride the wave." With this, we become eternal players in an eternal game. The difference, however, is that there is no stress and no strife when we are in sync with the patterns of nature. When we stop putting in chaotic noise, we can peacefully listen to *and dance with* the orchestra of all Creation. *It* moves us, *it* drives our action, and *it* becomes the guiding force for all our motives in goodness and in grace.

However, like the surfer who sees a wave coming, we have to paddle hard sometimes to catch it. Once we do, though, it is a great ride. We catch the tailwind, and it is smooth sailing from there.

So, where we go from here is obvious. We create the environment for our personal growth and healing, and we do so starting *right now*. There are a number of action steps that are important, and the follow-through of these is what makes or breaks an individual practice. Individual participation is where the rubber hits the road. With this in mind, we have covered a variety of topics in this book. In part II, we were introduced to highly effective practices to help us reconcile our energy losses and to correct the imbalances in our field. In our lives, we have spent a lot of time getting into a real mess, and it is going to take a number of steps to clean it up. Not to worry. We already know what we need to know for this stage, and we have the tools available to fix it. Now comes the practice.

I have found that after several years of dedicated training, the one thing that helps build the zhi, or the power of intention, better than anything is the practice of *gongs*. These gongs are personal agreements or rituals that we commit ourselves to in order to push our practice forward. We will learn about these at the end of this chapter, but it is first important to get a more global view of the action we need to take. This action involves looking at the world around us and our relationship to the notion of global citizenry. We need the Earth, and we need to create a healthy environment for cohabitation so that we have the necessary foundations for our practice.

Global Green Citizenry

In the Creation myth of the ancient Gnostic tradition, the planet Earth was formed when the Goddess Sophia "morphs into terrestrial form, becoming a planet herself, but an organic one, sentient and aware: the earth. . . . The terrestrial globe solidifies and life arises in rampant forms. . . . Sophia awakens to the world of her solitary dreaming, the template of the Anthropos and proceeds to live out a divine experiment: the unfolding of human novelty."[1] This becomes the basis of the Gnostic understanding of reality and the story of Creation, which, in this version, speaks of a sentient being from the center of the galaxy who comes out to the galactic arms in order to experiment with how life can emanate through her dream. Human beings, in the Gnostic understanding of reality, are the living acting agents of the "emanation" of Divinity, which comes to us *through* our connection with Sophia—the planet Earth. We are to co-create and evolve together because we are intimately tied to one another. This story is an important counterpoint to the Judeo-Christian version that places us in *dominion* over the Earth and that makes an important distinction that attributes Divinity as coming from above somewhere. This more Western version gives Divinity a characteristic *male* voice and, by deduction, places the feminine in an inferior position.

What we have learned about Taoism can come in and apply the magic of this rational way of looking at life to our Western notion of Divinity. A yang male god alone is a fundamental state of imbalance. There can be no yang without yin, and anything other than a perfect balance of the two cannot speak for the Ultimate Source (call it whatever you'd like). The fundamental split of yin and yang marks the birth of movement through separation, the birth of distinction and classification, duality as opposed to unity. Having a fundamentally male-oriented view of Divinity in the West, in my opinion, is a major contributor to the way we see ourselves, the way we see our surroundings, and, as a consequence, the way we relate to Mother Earth. Our imbalanced grasp of the Highest Aspect—or the Holiest of Holies, if you like—has created a cultural imbalance that has passively *allowed* for the raping of the Earth and the destruction of our ecosystem.

We measure progress not by how we cohabitate but by how well we can amass resources and pull "commodities" out of the natural environment. This way of thinking makes it perfectly okay to tear through a forest to pull out timber or to blast through a beautiful hillside to pull out coal. We draw fences and fight over terrain as if we own Her, as if She belongs to us, as opposed to the Native American view, which is the opposite: *we belong to Her.* We are in a symbiotic relationship with the planet. She needs us to evolve and wake up into fully sentient Light Bodies, and we need Her as a nurturing home. The magnetic field of the planet supports all life, and the myriad life-forms all around us create a web of interconnected energy fields that keep us connected to all life. They remind us of our birthright. To lose this connection by allowing mass extinctions to occur would be catastrophic for our species.

That being said, we do have certain needs, and coal is currently what keeps our houses warm. A balanced approach to development is the Taoist way. More innovation in technologies can allow us to harness the sun's energy, along with wind and geothermal, and make coal and oil extraction a thing of the past. The use of hyperdimensional physics, toroidal fields, and tapping into zero-point energy are not even conversations on the table yet (for political reasons—if we only knew the truth!), but they certainly should be.

In the postmodern era in which we live, it becomes important for us to really put away the dividing lines of nation-states and act together as a species in defense of our natural habitat. Lack of fresh water, overproduction of sewage, strip mining, desertification due to global warming, pollution in the seas, overfishing, deforestation, and overpopulation are issues that affect *all of us*. The distinct parts make up the whole, and if we all carry on thinking that we are the "chosen people," we will continue to draw our lines and fight over resources until it is too late. This idea takes us back to the notion of "enlightened citizenry."

Being truly enlightened means waking up, dispelling the clouds of the shadow trances in our heads, and seeing the world for what it truly is. Before these dark ages, the tribal units of our ancestors would hold the shamans or the wise men and women in the highest regard and follow their lead, as they were the clearest and most enlightened in the group. They were the leaders because of their wisdom. The return to enlightened citizenry requires the obvious substrate: *enlightened people*. It is up to us to wake up and take an active role in the happenings of our global policies, and it is up to us to ensure a safe and healthy future for our generations to come.

Green Economy

The notion of "money is evil" has hindered the spiritual community for decades and has kept the power in the hands of the ruling elite, who created the monetary system. By being part of a system that plays by those rules, many spiritually inclined people have shied away from "worldly" pursuits and have "hermitted" away into smaller communities that don't play on the main stage of global economics and politics. Just look where that has gotten us. Silence does not get you anywhere in a democratic system. Being duped into a two-party system run by the same corporate interests smells like an oligarchy, not a democracy. Actually, when corporate interests *become* the state interest, we move into fascism. Democracy is supposed to be a government for the people by the people, and we must exercise our rights as citizens. For too long now, the environment has been abused and damaged by the steady march of industry and the "advancement" of our species. But we now have the ability to do something about it; frankly, this is really our last chance before we forfeit our place as the "stewards" of the Garden. It is critically important for us to understand that *we vote with our dollars*. We are the consumers who drive the global economic system. We are the individual units who make up the whole. Each of us is a *critical* piece to the puzzle, and our direct and personal involvement in being part of the solution is absolutely necessary for the tide to turn in our race against humanmade global warming.

The more we sync up with the patterns of nature, the more we co-evolve with Sophia, the more we make right the conditions of the "fall" and the closer we come to restoring the Garden for our children's children. Here are some basic guidelines for being an active participant in the new green economy:

- Buy local organic produce from trusted sources.

- Get into a gas-efficient or electric car.

- Try to take public transportation, ride a bike, or carpool at least once a week.

- Check for leaks in the insulation of your house.

- No more bottled water! Buy a glass or stainless steel container and use a home filter.

- Change all your personal-care products to healthy ones that are made by reputable companies that don't conduct animal testing (or poison you).

- Cut out fast food from your diet; eating fast food supports unhealthy grazing practices.

- Use bamboo and other fast-growing trees for wood.

- Invest in green funds and green companies that include transparency in their corporate models.

- Spend your money on ideas and concepts that enrich your life. Cut down on the things that you don't need, and invest in experiences and growth-oriented endeavors.

These are just a few suggestions. Start today!

I feel that it is entirely appropriate to hold a vision for our future that performs major changes within one generation. So many policies lag in the United States because lawmakers can't risk signing on to anything that will make their constituents lose jobs. This is why we have an enormous military budget to this day. The arms makers provide hundreds of thousands of jobs in America, and nobody wants to risk messing with these, so we let the ball keep rolling. The problem with this is that we need to always have some armed conflicts going on somewhere in the world to *justify* these budgets. This leads to a foreign policy that helps provoke these conflicts. We somehow always need an enemy. We either let them blast each other and supply them with arms, or we put in a puppet and then go in to depose him a few years later. Polarity consciousness loves the good guy–bad guy paradigm or, worse, cowboy and Indian. We are culturally under this powerful trance. It is up to us to literally *create* a new economy that is green, healthy, life-affirming, and prosperous. Waiting for someone else to do it will get us all killed. We are the people we have been waiting for! Together, we can create a new medium of exchange that supports healthy lifestyles and green policies. We can strive to regain our place of cohabitation with the Earth and pursue more important goals of self-cultivation, illumination, the development of our Light Bodies, and, in short, our continued evolution into *Homo luminous*. The dark dream ends here.

A Taoist Perspective on Politics

As mentioned before, an excellent example of the polarization of our mind is reflected in the U.S. political system. You are either red or blue, for taxes or against them, an imperialist or an isolationist, pro-life or pro-choice. This simplistic approach to political discourse reflects the insanity of our times and the state of our collective consciousness. First of all, enlightened citizenry begins with awareness. This means we need to be *awake* enough to participate in our political processes. The people running the show now are puppeteers with specific economic interests who are looking out for their own constituents. It seems that the planet and the environment have taken all the flak for this, and we have suffered the loss of many ecosystems accordingly. Cohabitation with the various life-forms on the planet should take an important role in the future of politics, as biodiversity is a key element in the health of our overall ecosystem. Let us take a quick look at the big picture of where this is all going.

The accumulation—or, better yet, the "creation"—of wealth is something we take for granted in a capitalistic system. It has to be this way or else it's "communist," and that's evil. Again, polarity. This black-and-white classification of concepts is ingenious because it appeals to the primitive shadow-inspired trances in our consciousness, which invoke archetypal responses one way or another. It is the perfect tool of the puppeteer and has been used effectively for too long. At the end of the day, we all need to eat, we all want to enjoy our families, we all need water, and we'd all like to peacefully coexist in a beautiful natural environment, right? Okay, that means we need a medium of exchange to trade goods and services. Clams and beads were fine for hundreds of thousands of years, and then gold took over. The global bankers went out of their way to pull us off the gold standard in the early 1900s, so now all we're left with is a made-up "currency" that is printed by the

Federal Reserve System and that acts as legal tender. Actually, the Fed "lends" this money to our government, and we then pay it back with interest for years to come. (That's an idea beyond the scope of this book, but many sources offer more about this.) We then have a more "stable" economy where a bunch of cocky, twenty-four-year-olds who just got recruited onto Wall Street can dream up creative investment vehicles that make amazing amounts of money (for them) and gain them worldly power because of this. One day, the whole mess starts to collapse, and now, we stand here looking at this whole thing, not realizing that it is all a joke. It is a made-up system of value that we have created so that we can all get along and have a medium of exchange.

So, who determines the value? *We do.* Again, we vote with our dollars, and we vote our elected officials into office. The onus is on *us* to effectively steer the economy where we want it to go and to create healthy vehicles that make the world a better place. Invest your money with people and companies that are doing good things. Your money is nothing more than stored-up energy or credit that we use for trade. Society or markets establish this value, and we spend it accordingly. Do you value your energy and your life force? Do you value your time and your hard work? Do you care about the future of the planet and our species? Well, then, be more selective about where you put your energy! It is time to wake up and take ownership of our citizenry. We can only be leveraged and manipulated when we are asleep. It is time to wake up.

Let's Lay Out a Plan

We've covered a lot in this book, and now it is time to zip it all up together. A practice is only as good as its implementation, and there is only one person who can sit in that saddle: *you.* At this point, we know what the problem is and how we got into this mess.

I've outlined a number of practices here, all of which are helpful and all of which should be practiced regularly by you. I realize that you are not living in a monastery right now and that you have duties and obligations in your world. In the Taoist tradition, there are two main branches: Mountain Taoists and Fire Taoists.

The Mountain variety live up in the secluded enclaves of distant, nearly inaccessible ranges and lead lives of rigorous regimented practice and ritual observation. This is a very dedicated lifestyle that is a fast track to clearing obstructions in our fields; it gives us plenty of time each day to work on our Light Body. Less than 1 percent of the people I know have the luxury of living this lifestyle right now.

The Fire Taoists are the ones who live among the people. They are the ones who hold worldly professions but are committed to their practice and their energetic cultivation. They make their daily life and their interactions the basis of their qi gong. The world is their practice, and they diligently work on turning the daily "lead" of experience into the "gold" of realization and illumination both inside themselves and in the world around them as a reflection of their inner realization. These are the people the world needs right now. For every monk holding the light up in the mountains, we need ten thousand of us performing the Great Work right here in the society where we reside. There is no Garden apart from where we live; it's all One. This leaves us with the empowering knowledge that we are in a unique position to evolve and practice right here in our current lives, without shaving our heads or getting into a funny wardrobe. In fact, we needn't cling to any image. Let's just do the work.

This does not, however, preclude us from spending some time in nature, especially at first. Resonant tuning with the pure vibrations of nature is critical for us to calibrate to the energy curve of the Great Tao. Once we do so, we can continue to practice and cultivate that energy, maintaining our natural state and taking that into our daily lives. I personally take a minimum of a couple hikes per week. I call it "gathering the nectar," and I feel that it is an extremely rejuvenating practice. This is all part of the life of a Fire Taoist.

How to Begin Your Own Practice

Let's now summarize the whole battery of practices we have learned in this book and, more important, create a definitive *personal* plan to begin your own practice and start the Great Work. To keep it simple and digestible, I have outlined the major points under each category from this chapter. For further information, please refer to part II. It is important to remember that much of the information shared with you here was kept secret and was extremely coveted for thousands of years. It took me decades of diligent study and practice to reach the higher levels of these practices, many of which I have shared with you in this book. I'm not saying this because I'm fishing for applause; what I am interested in is imparting the tremendous *value* of what you've learned. I believe that times have changed. Know this: there is an entire brotherhood and sisterhood of people who are dedicated to *your growth* and your enlightenment. They are all committed to helping you achieve liberation and the fulfillment of your potential.

PHYSICAL PRACTICE

As mentioned earlier, the health of the physical vehicle is the underlying basis of this entire practice. Negligence of the body will deter your ultimate growth and keep you from developing the correct awareness of the Tao within you. The four major aspects of this practice are

- Diet
- Exercise
- Sleep
- Mindset

Review chapter 5 for a discussion about each of these.

QI GONG

The practices outlined in chapter 7 are designed to build a strong foundation in your energy field and help enhance the flow of your wei (defensive) qi and your ying (nutritive) qi. Altogether, to do all three would take just under forty-five minutes per day. If this is too much to start with, try doing one or two a day and *cycling* between them on different days. This will allow you to grow and develop the different skills and to fortify different aspects of your energy field as you go.

Daily practice of qi gong is essential, as it is the fastest way to clear your energy field and to dispel shadow energy charge. It frees up the underlying power you need to really delve into the Great Work. Again, the first exercise is available to view at SoundsTrue.com/inner-alchemy/bonus. I feel that in this modern age, there is no point in trying to learn moving exercises from a book. Watch the video and learn the exercise. The other two are in the book because they are static postures that can be captured in pictures.

The first hundred days of your practice are incredibly important. This is what is going to burn in a good habit and start the awakening process. I highly advise you to commit to a schedule you can uphold and to practice this daily.

MENTAL PRACTICE

The mental practice will function as the central "operating system" for your mind for years to come. Constantly asking yourself, "What am I doing right now?" is a conscious act of injecting self-awareness into the dreamy sleep of your unconscious days. With continued practice, you will begin to feel the freedom and liberation of simply *being*, instead of constantly doing and reacting. You can't feed your shadows when you do nothing; better yet, you can finally hear the undertones of your superconsciousness through your DNA when you finally stop "jumping in" with your incessant mental activities.

EMOTIONAL PRACTICE

The cleansing of emotional attachments is an incredibly liberating practice that frees up enormous reserves of energy. Emotions are *very* powerful and, when repressed, can compound into an explosive force. Learning to harmonize your emotional currents is critical. It is important to note that emotions are perfectly natural expressions that we all have to events. It is the imbalanced state of these emotions that creates suffering. If you allow them to naturally come and go, they are raw and real, and they are the very flavors of life. It is important to remember this, because there is nothing wrong with passion. Naturally emerging desires are a huge catalyst for growth, evolution, and change. The imbalanced reflection of your aversions and cravings is what causes the trouble and brings on your suffering.

The emotional cleansing practices in chapter 9 are very helpful and liberating. You will want to take some time at first to sit with these practices and get the hang of them. As with the mental practice, these tools should simply get burned into your subconscious mind and be running all day, almost like a virus scanner in a computer. You should program your subconscious mind to smooth out and heal imbalanced emotional charge as it comes up.

As you practice the mental awareness techniques, it will become obvious when you are getting carried away with an emotional charge. When you find this, you can, first of all, stop engaging in it any further (mental practice). Having illuminated it with your conscious mind, you can then proceed to heal it with the emotional practices you have learned. You can then return to your mental scanning and relaxation. As things pop up, forgive, heal, and clean the energies. Don't get frustrated—you have *years'* worth of stuff that you will start becoming aware of, and it'll take some time to heal and clear it all. You will eventually feel a thousand pounds lighter on the other side and will wonder how you ever lived carrying all of that "lead" around!

SPIRITUAL PRACTICE

We went over a number of very helpful techniques in chapter 10, many of which take some time to perform. I have shared these techniques to serve as a battery of tools at your disposal to continually clean and purify your energy field. Once you gain a visceral understanding of what it is you are truly doing, you'll be so enthused and excited to do this work that TV will be a thing of the past for you. There is nothing more amazing than the feeling of being totally clear of "gunk" and being able to simply be, see, and hear the love of the universe coursing through you. There is nothing left to do at this point. You are fully complete and have no wants. You are in ecstasy, just elated to be alive. This feeling is your birthright, and getting there is not an addition process. The more you *subtract*, the closer you come to Source. The more you cleanse and heal, the more whole you become. There is less of "you" and yet all of you.

Take your time and cycle through all of these practices, and you will find a rhythm that makes sense for you in your lifestyle. Do a minimum of one of these per week. Especially at first, be sure to take a number of dedicated acts of self-love to break out of your trance and wake up to the alchemical process. The task at hand is waiting for you, but you have to *see* the benefits before you fall back asleep.

MANIFESTATION PRACTICE

The manifestation practice becomes an important part of our work in that it allows us to understand the mechanism through which we can create the exact surroundings and circumstances we need in order to perform the Great Work. When we get a sense of how to silence our reactive mind and how to stop feeding energy into our shadows, we will have a clear channel for superconsciousness to fuse with our subconsciousness and guide us effortlessly in life. We can also learn to plant mental seeds via our self-consciousness directly into our subconsciousness to optimize our life and help quicken the healing process. We can learn to use this manifestation process to gain a profound understanding of our critically important role in the universe. It empowers us to shine the light of awareness on the shadows that house our mental, emotional, physical, and spiritual afflictions. A critical piece of the puzzle is learning the rules by which the universe operates and becoming a master of this knowledge.

The manifestation practice is based on an *understanding* of reality. Once we get a sense of how it is that things operate in our universe, we are empowered to play a more active role in the embedding of our own subconscious mind. More important, we then learn to "get out of the way" and let the currents of the Great Tao (or the Voice of God or whatever you want to call it) speak directly to us and guide our actions in life. We learn to move naturally with the waves of Creation and become co-creators.

To build this understanding into your daily life, it is important to pick a certain set of suggestions or goals that you would like to program into your subconsciousness and then do so on a daily basis in a "gong" (described below). You can learn to simultaneously listen to superconsciousness and program subconsciousness. Work on creating a set of reasonable goals and beliefs you would like to adopt. You can also set thirty-, sixty-, and hundred-day goals for your gong and reinforce them daily. I highly recommend using these tools, as they will help solidify your intention and focus your attention on your personal goals.

The Hundred-Day Gong

A gong in Chinese is a designated amount of time that you allot to perform a specific task daily. For example, knowing that it takes at least ninety days for a particular good habit to "burn into" your nervous system, I have found that the hundred-day gong is the most appropriate length to practice. This means that you pick a particular practice (or set of practices) and designate them as your gong, and you diligently practice them *every day* for one hundred days, without fail. This means that if you miss a day, even if it's day ninety-nine, you start over. Not only does this build resolve, it also forces you to wake up and pay attention to your day-to-day routines. It is incredibly painful when you miss day forty-six, for instance (I did!), and have to start over. At first you try to make excuses to yourself about how it was okay and how you'll just keep going, but then, a deal is a deal . . . you start over. Next round, you pay attention! It is a wonderful way of not only building focus and determination but also ensuring that you train regularly. It is a dedicated act of self-love that snaps you out of your daily trance and brings the light of awareness to your consciousness. The more you practice, the more you wake up and the better off you are.

I do these gongs all the time in my personal life and development. I set goals for myself for the next hundred days (physical, mental, spiritual), I look at them daily, and I reinforce my subconscious mind every day for those hundred days. When it is over, I assess where I am, and I take a few days of introspection and meditation before I set my next gong. In essence, I allow my superconscious mind to guide me into the next series of programs for the subconscious mind. This is a wonderful method for bringing the self-conscious mind into the equation and tying all aspects together, harmonizing yin and yang.

Depending on how dedicated you are and where you think you'd like to start, you can begin with something simple, like one qi gong set for starters, and do that for a hundred days. Or you can get far more involved. I usually have eight exercises or meditations per day in a given gong, but that's me; I've been a monk. Start where you feel like you can *realistically* manage it with your current time allowances and get the first hundred days under your belt. I assure you that afterward, you will do more of them and add more goals and practices as you go along.

This practice *really* helps get you on track and creates an environment for growth and personal development that is self-inspired and easy to follow. I've led thousands of people through gongs over the years and have seen people reverse diabetes, lose fifty pounds, increase their income tenfold, and find happiness. It's all about developing new micro habits and changing for the better every day. It's important to get a "win" early on with a reasonable gong that you can follow through with. Over time, you'll get better and be able to take bigger "bites."

Let's look at a couple of sample gongs for you to consider for your first hundred days.

SAMPLE GONG 1   Practice all of these daily

- Silk Weaver's Exercise

- Shaolin Standing Form

- Triple Burner Exercise

- 10 minutes of emotional clearing daily

- 15 minutes of mental practice daily

- Minimum 30 minutes of exercise 5 days per week, with 2 recovery days

- Focus on manifestation

SAMPLE GONG 2   Practice all of these daily

- Alternate between one of the following daily:
  › Silk Weaver's Exercise
  › Shaolin Standing Form
  › Triple Burner Exercise

- 30 minutes (in one sitting) of emotional clearing once per week

- 10 minutes of mental practice daily

- Minimum 30 minutes of exercise 5 days per week, with 2 recovery days

- Focus on manifestation

Now that you have read this book, you are equipped with the tools to start your practice and work toward full liberation and the ignition of the Light Body. This is all abstract knowledge, however, unless you actually engage in the daily practice and work toward this end. I have been commissioned to share this information with you, and, more important, I am here to support you. You, *yes, you*, are a central piece to the growth and evolution of our species, and you play a critically vital role in this process. I am committed to your evolution and enlightenment and will support you along the way. The more people who wake up, the faster and easier this process will be, and the faster the world will become a better and better place.

CONCLUSION

You now have all the tools you need to get started on your alchemical path. You understand the science behind how your problems are created, and you understand how to stop creating these problems. You understand where all the energy you feel you lack has gone and how to reclaim it from your shadow. You understand the principles of manifestation and are now equipped with the tools and resources to reprogram your subconsciousness and tune into the inner voice of superconsciousness. You have learned about the Light Body and have been given the powerful tools for the commencement of your journey to this level of awakening and understanding. You have learned a lot. I would like to take this opportunity to drive home the most important concept in this book: *do not sell yourself short.*

You are amazing and a critically important part of the whole universe. Wake up from your trances and wake up to the present moment. Wake up to your power and wake up to your potential. You are so incredibly special, and you will never cease to be amazed once you embark on the alchemical journey. I have laid out the necessary steps for you and have put together a number of tools and resources to help you at all stages along your path; there are more on my websites: well.org and theurbanmonk.com. Now, it is time to take that step.

The word *Namaste* in Sanskrit means "The Light within me respectfully bows to the Light within you."

Welcome home and *Namaste.*

In Loving Service,
Pedram Shojai

NOTES

CHAPTER 1: THE FREE FLOW OF ENERGY

1. Rosalyn Bruyere, *Wheels of Light: Chakras, Auras, and the Healing Energy of the Body* (New York: Touchstone, 1994), 241.
2. Jim Robbins, *A Symphony in the Brain: The Evolution of the New Brain Wave Biofeedback* (New York: Atlantic Monthly Press, 2000).
3. Paul Demorest, "Dynamo Theory and Earth's Magnetic Field," May 21, 2001, pdfs.semanticscholar.org/351e/344c1a92e7f20a e3d419f37cef59117eecb8.pdf.
4. Fritjof Capra, *The Tao of Physics: An Exploration of the Parallels Between Modern Physics and Eastern Mysticism* (Boston: Shambhala, 2010), 209.
5. Benoit Mandelbrot, *The Fractal Geometry of Nature* (Boston: W.H. Freeman, 1982), 5.
6. Leonard Orr, *Breaking the Death Habit: The Science of Everlasting Life* (Berkeley, CA: Frog, 1998).

CHAPTER 2: THE NATURE OF SUFFERING

1. Drunvalo Melchizedek, *The Ancient Secret of the Flower of Life* (Flagstaff, AZ: Light Technology Publishing, 1999), 411–19.

CHAPTER 3: A LIFESTYLE IN BALANCE

1. Jim Loehr and Tony Schwartz, *The Power of Full Engagement: Managing Energy, Not Time, Is the Key to High Performance and Personal Renewal* (New York: Free Press, 2003).
2. Hans Selye, *Stress Without Distress* (Philadelphia: Lippincott Williams & Wilkins, 1974).
3. George Mastorakos, Maria Pavlatou, Evanthia Diamanti-Kandarakis, and George P. Chrousos, "Exercise and the Stress System," *Hormones (Athens)* 4, 2 (April/June 2005): 73–89.

4. Stefanie Kalus, Thomas Kneib, Axel Steiger, Florian Holsboer, and Alexander Yassouridis, "A New Strategy to Analyze Possible Association Structures Between Dynamic Nocturnal Hormone Activities and Sleep Alterations in Humans," *American Journal of Physiology* 296, 4 (2009): 1216–27.
5. Mastorakos, et al. "Exercise and the Stress System," 73–89.
6. Christopher Ingraham, "The American Commute Is Worse Today Than It's Ever Been," *The Washington Post*, February 22, 2017, washingtonpost.com/news/wonk/wp/2017/02/22 /the-american-commute-is-worse-today-than-its-ever -been/?utm_term=.ae6dadf1c1f1.
7. Candace Pert, *Molecules of Emotion: Why You Feel the Way You Feel* (New York: Scribner, 1997), 131–45.
8. Alfred Korzybski, *Science and Sanity: An Introduction to Non-Aristotlian Systems and General Semantics* (New York: Institute of General Semantics, 1933).
9. Juraj Kukolja, Christiane M. Thiel, Marcus Wilms, Shahram Mirzazade, and Gereon R. Fink, "Ageing-Related Changes of Neural Activity Associated with Spatial Contextual Memory," *Neurobiology of Aging* 30, 4 (2007): 630–45.

CHAPTER 4: BASIC TAOIST THEORY

1. Giovanni Maciocia, *Foundations of Chinese Medicine: A Comprehensive Text*, 3rd ed. (Edinburgh, Scotland: Elsevier, 2015).
2. David Shier, *Hole's Human Anatomy & Physiology*, 11th ed. (Chicago: Wm. C. Brown Publishers, 1996), 107–11.
3. John Lamb Lash, *Not in His Image: Gnostic Vision, Sacred Ecology, and the Future of Belief* (White River Junction, VT: Chelsea Green, 2006).

CHAPTER 5: TENDING TO THE PHYSICAL VEHICLE

1. Li Dong-Yuan and Yang Shou-Zhong, *Treatise on the Spleen and Stomach: A Translation of the Pei Wei Lun* trans. Bob Flaws (Boulder, CO: Blue Poppy Press, 1993).

2. Fereydoon Batmanghelidj, *Water for Health, for Healing, for Life: You're Not Sick, You're Thirsty* (New York: Warner Books, 2003).
3. Office of Disease Prevention and Health Promotion, "2015–2020 Dietary Guidelines for Americans," accessed October 9, 2017, health.gov/dietaryguidelines/2015/guidelines /appendix-1/#table-a1-1.
4. Order of Shaolin Ch'an, *The Shaolin Grandmasters' Text: History, Philosophy, and Gung Fu of Shaolin Ch'an* (Beaverton, OR: Order of Shaolin Ch'an, 2004).
5. Kalus, et al. "A New Strategy to Analyze Possible Association Structures between Dynamic Nocturnal Hormone Activities and Sleep Alterations in Humans," 1216–27.

CHAPTER 9: EMOTIONAL PRACTICE

1. Korzybski, *Science and Sanity.*

CHAPTER 10: SPIRITUAL PRACTICE

1. *I Ching: The Classic Chinese Oracle of Change* trans. Rudolf Ritsema and Stephen Karcher (Rockport, TX: Element, 1994).
2. John Davidson, unpublished manuscript (given only to abbots of the Tao Tan Pai lineage), 2000.
3. Orr, *Breaking the Death Habit.*
4. Masaru Emoto, *The Hidden Messages in Water* trans. David A. Thayne (New York: Atria, 2005).
5. Tom Brown, *The Way of the Scout: A Native American Path to Finding Spiritual Meaning in a Physical World* (New York: Berkeley Publishing, 1995).

CHAPTER 11: THE PREDATORY UNIVERSE

1. Anonymous, *Meditations on the Tarot: A Journey into Christian Hermeticism* trans. Robert Powell (New York: Penguin Putnam, 1993), 408.

2. Charles Baudelaire, "Le Joueur Généreux," *Le Spleen de Paris* (Paris: Michel Levy, 1869).

CHAPTER 12: THE TAO OF MANIFESTATION

1. Michael Joyce, Paul Anderson, Marco Montouri, Luciano Pietronero, and Francesco Sylos Labini, "Fractal Cosmology in an Open Universe," *Europhysics Letters* 50, 3 (2000), iopscience.iop.org/article/10.1209/epl/i2000-00285-3/meta.
2. Jeremy Narby, *The Cosmic Serpent: DNA and the Origins of Knowledge* (New York: Tarcher, 1998).
3. M. Rattemeyer, F.A. Popp, and W. Nagl, "Evidence of Photon Emission from DNA in Living Systems," *Naturwissenschaften* 68, 11 (1981): 572–73.
4. Chet C. Sherwood, Cheryl D. Stimpson, Mary Ann Raghanti, Derek E. Wildman, Monica Uddin, Lawrence I. Grossman, Morris Goodman, John C. Redmond, Christopher J. Bonar, Joseph M. Erwin, and Patrick R. Hof, "Evolution of Increased Glia-Neuron Ratios in the Human Frontal Cortex," *PNAS* 103, 37 (2006): 13606–11, pnas.org/content/103/37/13606.

CHAPTER 13: THE BIRTH OF THE LIGHT BODY

1. Alberto Villoldo, *Shaman, Healer, Sage: How to Heal Yourself and Others with the Energy Medicine of the Americas* (New York: Harmony Books, 2000).
2. Gerald Schueler and Betty Schueler, *Egyptian Magick: Enter the Body of Light and Travel the Magickal Universe* (St. Paul, MN: Llewellyn Publications, 1994), 26–28.
3. Chogyal Namkhai Norbu, *The Crystal and the Way of Light: Sutra, Tantra, and Dzogchen* ed. John Shane (Ithaca, NY: Snow Lion, 1999), 158.
4. Norbu, *The Crystal and the Way of Light*, 158–59.
5. Lu K'uan Yu, *Taoist Yoga: Alchemy and Immortality* (York Beach, ME: Samuel Weiser, 1973), 163–71.

6. Paramahansa Yogananda, *Autobiography of a Yogi* (Los Angeles: Self Realization Fellowship, 1953), 149.
7. Villoldo, *Shaman, Healer, Sage*, 48–49.
8. Adolphe Napoléon Didron, *Christian Iconography: Or, The History of Christian Art in the Middle Ages* (London: H.G. Bohn, 1851).
9. *The Book of Enoch* trans. George Henry Schodde (Andover, MA: Warren F. Draper, 1911).
10. Gerald Massey, *Luniolatry, Ancient and Modern: A Lecture,* (1887; repr. Whitefish, MT: Kessinger Publishing), 175–87.

CHAPTER 14: WHERE WE GO FROM HERE

1. Lash, *Not in His Image*, 160.

GLOSSARY

Alchemy   the ancient art of transmutation, which is the foundation of esoteric spiritual work. The premise is the transformation of lead to gold, which in the human experience is taken metaphorically as the refinement of our internal energy and our life's processes into coherent white light and full self-realization. This practice is the basis of our work here, and we return to this concept throughout the book.

Dantien   the energy reserve area where qi energies come together, gather, condense, and rarify. According to the ancient Taoists, there are three main dantiens along the central channel of the human body. The lower dantien is located three fingers below the navel and spans from the front of the body to the spine. The middle dantien is centered in the chest at the heart level. The upper dantien is located slightly above eye level in the center of the forehead. The lower dantien is the primary reserve center from which we breathe and cultivate energy during our qi gong practice. Each center needs to be cultivated slightly differently. They need to be unlocked in sequence to attain true enlightenment and liberation.

Defensive Qi   also called *wei qi*, this is the type of energy that circulates around the exterior of the body. It is in charge of protecting our systems from exterior attack. It can be likened to the functions of the immune system. It helps open and close pores on the skin and helps maintain smooth flow of energy along our exterior "force field." Healthy wei qi is critical for our practice to progress.

Energy Field   connotes the shell of energy surrounding our physical bodies. All life-forms have energy fields that tend to be the tangential reflection of the state of overall flow of energy throughout our systems. The purpose of the qi gong practitioner is to cultivate the flow and quality of this energy field to remove any blockages or impedance. The cleaner and clearer these fields are, the closer we are to Source energy, and the more power and grace can run through us.

Essence   also called "vitality," this is the level of energy or substance that represents the core genetic makeup of who we are. Our essence is tied to our sexuality and comes through to us from our parents. It is the reserve system or battery for the qi energy that runs through our bodies. It is to be guarded and cultivated by the advanced practitioner.

Five Elements   the Chinese medical system breaks all of reality down into five flavors or elements of emanation: fire, wood, water, metal, and earth. Each element represents the movement of energy in nature through the cycles of yin and yang. Each has particular correspondences with colors, sounds, flavors, emotions, internal organs, and tissues.

Food Qi   this is the energy we extract from food. It mixes with the energy we draw from the air and then pools in the center of the chest to become usable in a metabolic sense.

Gathering Qi   this energy forms when air and food qi combine in the chest. With the help of the original qi coming from the kidney essence, this form of energy makes the true qi, which then feeds into the body's nutritive and defensive energies.

Gong   a designated set of activities that we sign up to do for a set period. These are conscious acts of self-love and dedicated attention to self-care. The typical gong recommended in this book is for one hundred days, as it takes at least ninety days to establish behavioral re-patterning. It is important to choose a reasonable set of practices to perform daily and not to miss a day for one hundred days. Any slip-up means you have to start over at day one. This helps develop focus and willpower while creating good habits and enhancing the overall health of the system.

Homo luminous   coined by Inca scholar and teacher Alberto Villoldo, this state represents the next level of evolution of the human species from *Homo sapiens.* The premise is that our next level of growth bridges into self-discovery and the understanding of the energetic matrix around us. From here we wake up and activate our Light Body, literally evolving into the next stage of our growth.

Hun the ethereal soul that is housed in the liver and is attributed to the wood element. The hun is responsible for the body's connection to spirit. It can be best described as the astral body. If it is not properly rooted and anchored in the liver blood, we can feel restless at night and have strange dreams. An unrooted hun also leads to a loss of direction in life. According to Taoist tradition, upon dying this soul is released upward to heaven.

I Ching the ancient Chinese book of changes. This miraculous work breaks all reality into a series of trigrams and hexagrams based on a binary linear code of yin and yang expressions. A solid line is yang, and a broken one is yin. These trigrams and hexagrams code into sixty-four different possibilities, which mirror our genetic code and describe all emanations of reality. The book is also used to cast fortunes and foretell the future through divination.

Jing also called "vitality" or "essence," this is the level of energy or substance that represents the core genetic makeup of who we are. Our essence is tied to our sexuality and comes through to us from our parents. It is the reserve system or battery for the qi energy that runs through our bodies. It is to be guarded and cultivated by the advanced practitioner. Jing, qi, and shen are considered the Three Treasures of the body and are to be cultivated daily.

Kung Fu the ancient martial art of China practiced by thousands of monks for centuries. The literal translation is "hard work" or "eat bitter." Kung fu is grounded in deep qi gong knowledge and uses the meridian system of qi flow to potentiate power and direct lethal strikes. Many of the qi gong systems we study in this book are grounded in kung fu, as the two were inextricable in the temple systems through which they were preserved. Deep kung fu stances are important to cultivate in order to ground our energy and harness our internal power via qi gong.

Light Body the luminous glowing field of energy that is activated once we have properly cultivated and refined our qi. There are Light Body traditions all over the world, and they all allude to a luminous glowing field around the physical body. Once activated, practitioners can slough off their physical body and maintain continuous consciousness because they are free from the cycle of birth and rebirth. Light Body cultivation becomes the central theme of our work once we have removed blockages in our energy fields and are ready for the transformation of our "lead" to this spiritual "gold."

Meridians the network of channels or pathways for the flow of qi energy through the human body. There are twelve primary meridians, along with eight "extraordinary" ones. These meridians represent each of the internal organs, along with certain metabolic functions and psychic channels. The smooth flow of qi along these meridians is critical for the maintenance of good health and vitality.

Nei Gong the internal form of qi gong that focuses on the alchemical aspects of the practice. Here, the practitioner gathers and concentrates energy in the dantiens and works to refine and cultivate awareness. The expansion and refinement of consciousness are natural components to this practice. As the Light Body is activated, the flow and coherence of energy and light are optimized and tuned to Source energy.

Nutritive Qi after the energy of food and air come together, they are infused with the original qi derived from the essence. This true qi then differentiates into nutritive and defensive qi. The nutritive qi is the raw energy the body uses to maintain, heal, and restore the internal organs. This is the energy we run off for our day-to-day needs. It must be maintained and cultivated so that we are in relative abundance so as to not deprive our vital organs of the energy they need to thrive.

Original Qi this is the energy derived from the essence that is stored in the kidneys. This vital energy comes from our genetic "bank account" and is used to infuse the energy we derive from food and air. The original qi is stored in the lower dantien and is a vital force in our overall energy system. In our qi gong, we work to nourish, maintain, and maximize the original qi by nourishing the essence and optimizing efficiency in the system.

Po   the "corporeal" soul that is housed in the lungs. This is the most physical and material part of a human's soul and is intimately connected with our breathing. Author Giovanni Maciocia calls it "a direct manifestation of the breath of life." The po returns to the earth upon our death and is related to constrained feelings of sadness and grief.

Prana   the vital energy that is tied to breath in the Indian yogic system. The prana flows through nadi, or channels of energy (much like the meridians in the Chinese system) throughout the body. There are nodes of greater concentration, and the goal of the practitioner is to breathe awareness and attention to blocked regions in the body to allow the prana to flow in and heal.

Qi   the vital energy that circulates through all life. It is the currency of exchange among all life-forms and is the moving aspect of sentience. Its refined form is spirit, and its substantiated form is essence. Qi circulates through meridians (energy pathways) throughout the human body and is attained through air and food. The state of our qi flow directly influences our health. Qi is to be cultivated, refined, and moved in order for us to wake up. Stagnant qi is the cause of many disease processes.

Qi Gong   the ancient practice of energy cultivation from China. Literally translated as "energy work," this practice, along with meditation, is the foundation of most temple arts. Kung fu, tai chi, and Chinese medicine all have forms of qi gong, as the cultivation of the vital qi energy in our systems is tantamount to the activation of our Light Body.

Shaolin   the famous Chinese school of martial arts and Buddhism. Shaolin was an existing Buddhist temple before being visited by Bodhidharma, the famous monk who transformed the school with his introduction of qi gong. Bodhidharma created the famous "warrior monks" of the Shaolin Temple and trained them to be the defenders of good in ancient China.

Shen   the spirit, which is housed in our hearts. Shen is one of the Three Treasures in Chinese medicine (qi/energy, jing/essence, and shen/spirit). Shen is the awakened understanding of who we truly are and the manifestation of that existence in our bodies. We are to cultivate and refine our shen and our awareness through our practice of qi gong and meditation. A clear mind leads to clear shen, and clear shen leads to enlightenment.

Shen Gong   the practice of cultivating spirit or shen. This practice is not to be confused with devotional prayer, because the Chinese translation here uses the meaning of "mind" for shen. In this light, shen gong is the cultivation of psychic perception, ESP, clairvoyance, and other mental powers through specific practices. One of the early shen gong exercises a student learns is to see the energy between their fingertips in a certain stance or to see the aura of a person. Shen gong is useful for healers and is a powerful tool for awareness, but should be only practiced as part of an overall balanced curriculum.

Tai Chi Chuan   a martial art that is become very popular in the West. Translated as "the grand ultimate fist," it is revered for its slow movements and graceful appearance. Done correctly, tai chi is a sophisticated martial art with an underlying foundation in qi gong and energy awareness. In essence, it allows the practitioner to *become* the stage wherein yin and yang dance in their interplay. Known for its many health benefits, tai chi has become quite a hit in the United States.

Tantra   the ancient spiritual practice of energy cultivation through sexual co-stimulation. Tantra is a high art wherein the practitioners tap into their powerful essence energy and use qi and shen to fuse, ignite, and raise the *kundalini* energy, which is stored at the base of the spine. It is extremely powerful and should be done carefully. Done right, Tantra liberates our minds from sexual aberration and brings forth deep understanding of our essential divine nature.

Taoism   the ancient Chinese philosophy of balance and harmony with nature. Based on the principle of the mutual enhancement and interaction of yin (passive) and yang (active) forces in nature, Taoism teaches us to find balance in every facet of our lives. There is also religious Taoism, which bridges into the various deity worship traditions of ancient China. Note: This religious Taoism is not the variety represented in this book. In this book, we are talking about the life philosophy or mastery as developed by the ancient Taoist sages, Lao Tzu and Chuang Tzu. We use those as our base and work to develop a modern understanding of them as applied to today's world.

Wei Gong   the form of qi gong energy cultivation that works on the wei qi, or external defensive energy of the body. Wei gong helps bolster immunity and protects the body from external pathogens. It is always important to have some wei gong practice in our regimen, as this becomes a policy of health *assurance* in a world where health *insurance* does so little.

Yang   the active expression of the universe/Tao, which is the balanced counterpart to the yin expression. In the example of hot and cold, hot would be the yang attribute.

Yi   the central intellect or the mind, which is housed in the spleen. This is the self-conscious aspect of the mind where we must learn to integrate and assimilate information. A calm mind and a healthy connection with one's superconscious aspects, combined with a healthy relationship with one's subconscious mind, are all critical facets of having a healthy yi.

Yin   the passive expression of the universe/Tao, which is the balanced counterpart to the yang expression. In the example of hot and cold, cold would be the yin attribute.

Yoga   the ancient Indian art of body/mind/spirit cultivation. The word means "union," and it serves as an alchemical vehicle for the development of the Light Body. The yogi works to open blockages in the nadi (energy pathways/meridians) through breathing into specific postures, *asanas*, while cultivating awareness and relaxing into the body. Self-awareness and enlightenment are the ultimate goals of this sophisticated system. We see a very watered-down version in the West, but the essence of this practice is quite noble and is a true pathway toward liberation.

Zero-Point Energy   the amount of energy associated with the vacuum of empty space. This is predicted to be infinite, as it is the sum of the energy of all the subatomic particle interactions of the universe. Tapping into this field is the subject of much study in science. It has been proposed that ascended masters can tap into this field through their consciousness. It is important to note that, for decades, spiritualists have been jumping onto new nomenclature in physics as things are discovered. This term may not be what we are sensing or tapping into with our meditation practice, and traditional physicists would argue that, according to their theorems and equations, it is impossible. Bridging science and spirituality is an exciting field, and much work has to be done to clear up the semantic parallels.

Zhi   the willpower, which is housed in the kidneys. The zhi is the water element's "spirit" and is tantamount in our ongoing development. The zhi of the kidneys needs to work with the shen and attention of the heart for us to be present and awake. The serious student builds and cultivates zhi through practice (especially gongs) in order to step into their personal power. From here, their energy is properly activated, and the qi flow is robust and unblocked.

ACKNOWLEDGMENTS

To the loves of my life—Elmira, Sol, and Sophia. You are the light of my life, and I savor the moments we are together. I owe everything to my beloved parents, Farhad and Sonbol Shojai, who brought us to America in times of uncertainty. They were seeking a better future for their children and sacrificed everything they had in order to make that future a reality. The degree of selflessness and personal commitment to family, love, and mutual respect always served as the central foundation of my worldview and has helped me become the man I am today. I can never thank them enough for setting their own dreams aside in order for us to realize ours. They wanted a better world for me; in that light, the only way I know how to repay them is to make the world I have stepped into a better place—not just my neighborhood or my suburb, but the entire world through and through. Thanks to Farhad and Sonbol Shojai, I am committed to shining the light of love and realization through the shadows so that goodness reigns on Earth once again.

I would also like to thank my sister Shery, who has lovingly been by my side throughout the years and has always believed in me. Again, being surrounded by love and mutual respect is an honor that is not to be taken lightly.

There are also many teachers, masters, doctors, and friends to thank—too many to list them all. One, in particular, deserves a full salute—Grand Master Carl Totton. He has been my guide, friend, teacher, and mentor for many years. He has served as a major influence in my awakening and continued development. The world owes Sifu Totton immense gratitude for preserving the essence of the Chinese internal arts and for so openly sharing these secrets.

ABOUT THE AUTHOR

Pedram Shojai is a doctor of oriental medicine, a Taoist abbot, and *New York Times* best-selling author. He's an award-winning filmmaker, lecturer, and thought leader in the mind-body space. Pedram has transitioned from "ascetic" monk to "Urban Monk," as he's now a householder with a wife, two children, and a happy family life. He continues to work diligently to protect the environment and is a vocal advocate of conscious capitalism.

ABOUT SOUNDS TRUE

Sounds True is a multimedia publisher whose mission is to inspire and support personal transformation and spiritual awakening. Founded in 1985 and located in Boulder, Colorado, we work with many of the leading spiritual teachers, thinkers, healers, and visionary artists of our time. We strive with every title to preserve the essential "living wisdom" of the author or artist. It is our goal to create products that not only provide information to a reader or listener, but that also embody the quality of a wisdom transmission.

For those seeking genuine transformation, Sounds True is your trusted partner. At SoundsTrue.com you will find a wealth of free resources to support your journey, including exclusive weekly audio interviews, free downloads, interactive learning tools, and other special savings on all our titles.

To learn more, please visit SoundsTrue.com/freegifts or call us toll-free at 800.333.9185.

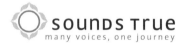